AIDS: SCIENTIFIC AND SOCIAL ISSUES

A Resource for Health Educators

AIDS: SCIENTIFIC AND SOCIAL ISSUES

A Resource for Health Educators

PETER AGGLETON, HILARY HOMANS,
JAN MOJSA, STUART WATSON AND
SIMON WATNEY

Faculty of Education & Community Studies
Bristol Polytechnic

Churchill Livingstone
Edinburgh London Melbourne and New York 1989

CHURCHILL LIVINGSTONE
Medical Division of Longman Group UK Limited

Distributed in the United States of America by
Churchill Livingstone Inc., 1560 Broadway, New York,
N.Y. 10036, and by associated companies, branches
and representatives throughout the world.

First published 1989
  Reprinted 1990

ISBN 0 443 04182 2

Produced by Longman Singapore Publishers (Pte) Ltd.
Printed in Singapore

Contents

The project team would like to thank all those who
have offered advice, support and encouragement
in the writing of this book. A detailed list of the
individuals and organisations who have helped in
this way can be found in the introductory
booklet to the *Learning About AIDS* package.

Introduction

The first cases of Acquired Immune Deficiency Syndrome (AIDS) were diagnosed in the early 1980s amongst young gay men resident in American cities such as San Francisco, Los Angeles, New York and Miami. Most of those affected were in their twenties or thirties, and were diagnosed with either a hitherto rare form of pneumonia called Pneumocystis carinii pneumonia, or a skin tumour known as Kaposi's sarcoma. Subsequently, AIDS has been diagnosed among haemophiliacs, injecting drug users, children, the recipients of blood transfusions, heterosexuals and bisexuals – indeed, amongst members of just about every social group into which people can be classified. At the time of writing (June 1988), the World Health Organization estimates that there are over 100,000 cases of AIDS worldwide, with between five and ten million others being infected by Human Immunodeficiency Virus (HIV), the virus which causes the syndrome. As yet, there is no vaccine to protect against infection, and neither is there a cure. Within this context, health education has been identified as the key with which to stop further infection. It has also been identified as the means for alleviating unreasonable fears and anxieties and reducing prejudice.

There are many different ways in which health education about HIV infection and AIDS can take place. These various styles of health education, or models of health education as they are sometimes called, differ from one another both in terms of their goals and their means. Some favour information-giving as a way of bringing about changes in the way individuals behave. Others advocate the use of more participatory forms of learning. Yet further approaches suggest that health education should aim to do more than bring about individual changes in behaviour. It should also seek to self-empower, to foster community development or to bring about far-reaching social change. As yet there is little consensus on these issues, but of one thing we can be certain – health educators will need to be well prepared when the focus of their work is on HIV infection and AIDS.

In writing this book, we have tried to satisfy two related sets of demands. First, it is a key resource for health educators using *Learning about AIDS* materials. In late 1986, work began at Bristol Polytechnic on a project supported by the Health Education Authority, the aims of which were to develop participatory strategies for use in adult education about HIV infection and AIDS. Interim health education materials from this project were produced and disseminated in mid-1987. Subsequently, a much more extended range of exercises has been developed. These make up the *Learning about AIDS* programme that is currently under dissemination in England.

Participatory styles of health education such as these require health educators to be well versed in the issues that can arise in connection with their work with different client groups. Whilst some may find they have easy access to the relevant medical, scientific and social science literature, others may find they have to rely on secondary sources for their information. Sadly, few books have been written with the needs of health educators specifically in mind. We have therefore put together background information relating to the medical, scientific and social issues that are likely to arise on *Learning about AIDS* courses.

We also hope this book will be a resource for health educators more generally. Teachers in schools and colleges may find it valuable as background material for their work with young people. Health Education Officers, Health Service Trainers, Health Advisers, Nurse Tutors and others may find it useful in connection with their work with health professionals. Trainers working in social services, youth and community education and the voluntary sector may feel more confident in their ability to examine the relevant issues after reading it, and those working in the private sector may find that it helps them prepare for the rather more focused kind of work that they may be asked to undertake.

In a book of this length, it is not possible to cover all the issues. Further references are therefore provided with each chapter and in the appendices that can be found at the end of the book. Nevertheless, we hope that health educators from all backgrounds will find this book useful as a review of current scientific, medical and social debates. If, after reading it, they feel more confident to tackle the issues raised by HIV infection and AIDS, our goals will have been achieved.

1.   Medical and scientific issues

1.1   WHAT IS AIDS?

AIDS stands for Acquired Immune Deficiency Syndrome – a medically defined condition first identified in the early 1980s among young gay men resident in New York and San Francisco. It has subsequently been diagnosed in a wide range of other settings. In Europe, North and South America, Asia and Australasia, those particularly affected at the present time include gay and bisexual men, haemophiliacs, injecting drug users, prostitutes and the recipients of blood transfusions and blood products. In some parts of sub-Saharan Africa, however, AIDS has been diagnosed more generally than this, and roughly equal numbers of women and men have been affected.

The original definition
Before Human Immunodeficiency Virus (HIV) was identified as the cause of AIDS and before tests were developed to detect the virus, AIDS was defined as a syndrome diagnosed by the *presence* of one or more very specific diseases that rarely affect people whose immune systems are working efficiently. These opportunistic diseases had to be present in the *absence* of all other possible causes of immune deficiency. Thus, if a person receiving immuno-suppressive medication contracted one of them, they would not be diagnosed as having AIDS.

The opportunistic diseases associated with AIDS were originally divided into two main types – infections and tumours. One particular infection, Pneumocystis carinii pneumonia (PCP), was identified early in the epidemic and still accounts for the majority of diagnoses made. Others were identified later and include toxoplasmosis, another protozoal infection, and crypto-coccosis, a fungal infection. Both of these affect the brain and central nervous system, the lungs and the heart. Other opportunistic infections include cytomegalovirus (CMV) infection affecting the lungs and nervous system, candida (yeast) infection affecting the lungs and oesophagus and cryptosporidium infection which causes persistent diarrhoea. Contrary to popular belief, people with AIDS are not more prone than others to infections such as the common cold (Figure 1).

Figure 1: *Opportunistic infections seen in AIDS*

PROTOZOAL INFECTIONS
Pneumocystis carinii
Toxoplasma gondii
Cryptosporidium species
Isospora species

BACTERIAL INFECTIONS
Mycobacterium tuberculosis
Mycobacterium avium-intracellulare
Mycobacterium kansasii/xenopi
Salmonella typhimurium
Shigella flexneri

FUNGAL INFECTIONS
Candida albicans
Cryptococcus neoformans

VIRAL INFECTIONS
Cytomegalovirus
Herpes simplex
Papova viruses (JC/SV-40)

Concurrent infection by a number of these pathogens is often seen in AIDS

Tumours identified by the original definition included Kaposi's sarcoma (KS), a normally rare kind of skin cancer which, in AIDS, can become widespread throughout the body, and lymphomas, particularly in the brain and central nervous system.

The current definition
More recently, it has become clear that brain disease in the absence of identifiable opportunistic infections or tumours can sometimes be found in people with AIDS, as can diseases of other organs including the heart, pancreas, lungs and gut. Brain disease is sometimes accompanied by meningitis and encephalopathy as well as behavioural changes, memory deficits and a loss of bodily co-ordination. Additionally, a virus (HIV) has now been identified as the cause of AIDS.

These two events led to the publication in 1987 of a revised definition of AIDS (CDC, 1987). As before, AIDS is diagnosed by the presence of one or more specific diseases in the absence of any other known cause of immune deficiency. However, the results of laboratory tests for HIV are now taken into account in making the diagnosis.

Where the test results are *unknown* or *inconclusive*, the identification of an opportunistic infection such as PCP or a tumour such as KS is sufficient for a diagnosis of AIDS, assuming there are no other causes of immune deficiency.

Where there is a *positive* test result, however, a wider range of diseases than hitherto can lead to the diagnosis of AIDS. These now include diseases such as encephalopathy and wasting, in addition to the opportunistic infections and tumours that were first associated with the syndrome.

Where there is a *negative* test result, and where other causes of immune deficiency have been ruled out, AIDS can still be diagnosed if the person has developed PCP or, if there is evidence of marked immune suppression, one of a limited number of other opportunistic diseases.

1.2 MEDICAL EXPLANATIONS

The current definition of AIDS therefore makes reference to the consequences of HIV infection. Nowadays, most doctors believe that HIV is the cause of AIDS, although this has not always been the case. In Europe and North America, suspicions were first aroused about a possible viral cause when it was noted that AIDS seemed to affect relatively discrete groups of people – gay and bisexual men, injecting drug users, haemophiliacs and so on.

In late 1983, a team of researchers working in Paris isolated a new virus from tissue from a gay man with persistently swollen lymph glands. They called the virus Lymphadenopathy Virus (LAV). Shortly after this, another research team working in the United States isolated a similar virus from a number of men with AIDS. They called this virus Human T-cell Lymphotropic Virus Type III (HTLV-III). In order to resolve the problem of terminology, this virus has subsequently been renamed Human Immunodeficiency Virus (HIV).

It is now widely accepted that HIV is the cause, not only of AIDS, but of a wide range of related conditions. These include acute HIV infection, Persistent Generalised Lymphadenopathy (PGL) and AIDS-Related Complex (ARC). Acute HIV infection takes the form of a glandular-fever-like illness lasting for a couple of weeks or so. Typically, the person experiences a fever, sore throat, headache, rash and general malaise. Not all who are infected experience this illness. PGL on the other hand takes the form of persistently swollen lymph nodes. These must be at least 1 cm in diameter and present for more than three months in two or more sites away from the groin for PGL to be diagnosed. Other causes for the swollen glands must of course be ruled out. The term ARC is usually used to describe a combination of symptoms including fever, night sweats, aches, fatigue, sickness and diarrhoea.

Many people with HIV infection show no symptoms, at least in the short term. Estimates vary depending on the group studied, but at the time of writing it is widely accepted that within five years of infection, 10–30% of people will develop AIDS and between 20–50% of others will develop PGL or ARC (WHO, 1988). Over a longer timescale than this, we do not know what proportion of infected people will develop AIDS.

A number of different theories have been put forward to explain how AIDS may develop in an infected individual. Most doctors currently believe that HIV is necessary and sufficient to cause AIDS. While this kind of explanation acknowledges that there can be many different consequences of HIV infection, it suggests that progression from one to another is likely to take place (Figure 2).

Figure 2: HIV as a necessary and sufficient cause of AIDS

HIV⟶ Asymptomatic⟶ Persistent————▶ AIDS-Related⟶ AIDS
        state   Generalised   Complex
                           Lymphadeno-   (ARC)
                           pathy (PGL)

Other doctors have argued that co-factors might be involved in progression from one state to another. One early report suggested that genetic factors might be involved here (Eales *et al*, 1987), although subsequent attempts to replicate the findings on which these claims were based have proved unsuccessful (Nixon *et al*, 1987), and the authors of the original study have since retracted or considerably modified their earlier claims (Eales *et al*, 1988).

On the other hand, there is evidence to suggest that subsequent infection by other sexually transmitted diseases may increase the likelihood that AIDS will develop in an HIV-infected person (Weber *et al*, 1986). It has also been suggested that pregnancy in a woman who is HIV positive may increase her risk of developing AIDS (Pinching & Jefferies, 1985), although this evidence too has been contested by other researchers (Ciraru-Vigneron *et al*, 1987).

Alternative explanations

As is the case with any new disease, scientific and medical opinions differ when it comes to explaining cause. Whilst one particular explanation may become widely accepted and become the orthodox view, there may also be other competing explanations. These are frequently regarded as 'crackpot' ideas by those who subscribe to mainstream opinion. Nevertheless, since they may well be encountered within the context of AIDS education, it is important to be aware of their existence.

When it comes to explaining AIDS, two differing kinds of alternative explanations exist. First, there are those that preceded the isolation and identification of HIV. One of these suggests that AIDS might be caused by an overloading of the immune system – perhaps through repeated infection by sexually transmitted diseases or by the excessive use of recreational drugs such as amyl and butyl nitrite, commonly called 'poppers' (Lauritsen, 1986). Then there is the view that a combination of co-factors may be needed for a person to develop AIDS. Early theories of this kind suggested that immune overload might re-activate earlier viral infections. In combination with one another, these might subsequently produce immune breakdown. Later theories like this suggest that HIV infection may be necessary but not sufficient to cause AIDS, co-factors being necessary for the development of the syndrome itself.

Second, there are explanations developed after the isolation and identification of HIV. Some of these suggest that HIV is an opportunistic infection which affects only those who are already immune compromised (Duesberg, 1987). According to this type of theory, an as yet unidentified agent may be the real cause of AIDS. Candidates for this include African Swine Fever Virus which causes fever, enlarged lymph nodes, skin lesions, immune modulated pneumonia and brain disease in pigs (Beldekas et al, 1986) and a new as yet unnamed virus isolated from people with AIDS (Lo, 1986).

1.3   THE HUMAN IMMUNE SYSTEM

Since AIDS results from a defect in the immune system, it is important to know something about immunity and how it works.

What is meant by immunity?

Immunity is the process by which the body is able to protect itself from infection and disease. Until recently, relatively little has been known about immunity – hence the existence of numerous lay theories which claim to explain the processes involved (see Chapter 4). In the last fifteen years, however, considerable advances have been made in our understanding of immunity and how it works.

Many different mechanisms are involved in immunity. Some of these involve physical barriers such as the skin and the mucous membranes. These safeguard against infection by a wide range of potentially harmful micro-organisms or germs. Other immune processes involve special chemical substances which can inactivate potentially harmful viruses and bacteria. Saliva, for example, contains substances which are capable of inactivating some viruses, and tears contain a substance called lysozyme which can deal with some bacteria (Figure 3).

Figure 3: Physical and chemical barriers providing immunity

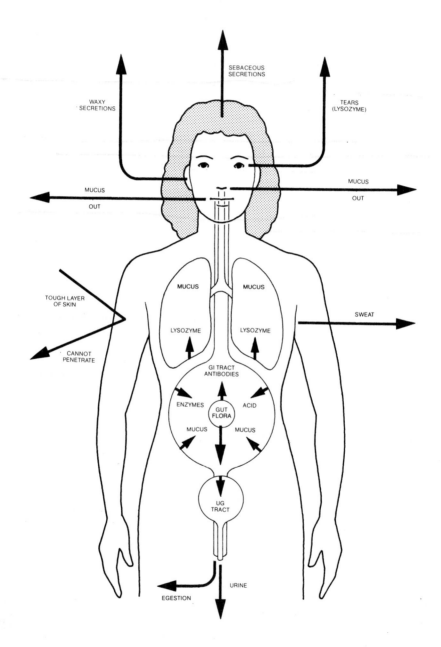

There are also more specific aspects of immunity. These generally involve specialised cells in the blood which deal with potentially harmful micro-organisms once they have entered the body. Some of these cells deal with the infecting micro-organisms directly whereas others do so by producing chemical substances known as *antibodies* which then neutralise the infection. These processes will be examined in detail later.

It is important to realise that the immune system is an active system. Its various components are at work night and day, detecting and dealing with numerous micro-organisms that might otherwise cause harm. Harmful micro-organisms, or *pathogens* as they are sometimes called, are all around. The fact that we do not normally worry about them shows how easy it is to take for granted the work that the immune system does in protecting us from them (Figure 4).

Figure 4: Some common pathogens

Bacteria   Bacteria are small single-celled organisms. There are many different kinds of bacteria. Some of the better-known bacteria cause sore throats, scarlet fever, gonorrhoea, tuberculosis and syphilis.

Viruses   Viruses are the smallest living things we know about. They are parasites and can only reproduce themselves inside the cells of another living organism. Some viruses live in animal cells and others in plant cells. Generally speaking, viruses are highly species specific – that is, they are attracted to and reproduce within the cells of only one organism. Common kinds of viruses include the influenza virus, the mumps and measles viruses and the herpes viruses.

Protozoa   Protozoa are single-celled animals and are able to withstand harsh conditions by developing into cysts. Diseases caused by protozoal infections include malaria, sleeping sickness and amoebic dysentery.

Fungi   Fungi are simple plants which lack chlorophyll and hence the ability to photosynthesise. Common fungal infections include ringworm and thrush.

But there is another reason why we need have little fear of many of the pathogens that surround us. This is because, in order for infection to take place, a *critical quantity* of that micro-organism must enter our bodies through a *critical route.* Contrary to popular belief, simply being in the presence of a pathogen is not sufficient for infection to occur. Germs rarely if ever spread through the air like a mist or infect us simply because we are in their vicinity. They have to enter the body by specific routes and in specific amounts for infection to take place (Figure 5). Medical and scientific understandings such as these contrast sharply with earlier theories about disease which suggested that diseases spread like a vapour through the air, affecting all who come into contact with them.

Figure 5: Some common means of virus transmission

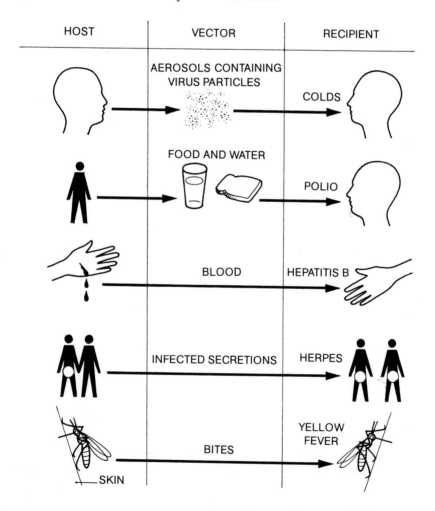

Specific resistance to disease

There are two different mechanisms involved in specific resistance, both of which involve white blood cells, *leucocytes*. The majority of white blood cells are *phagocytes*, generalists whose task it is to recognise, bind to and engulf a whole range of bacteria, viruses and other pathogens (Figure 6). Their work is supplemented, however, by a variety of more specialised white blood cells called *lymphocytes*, the most important types of which are B-cells and T-cells. These are manufactured in the bone marrow and the thymus gland respectively, hence their names.

Figure 6: A phagocyte engulfing a bacterium

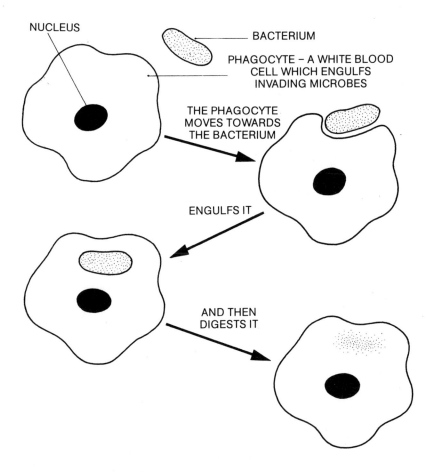

B-cells B-cells are particularly effective against infections caused by bacteria and viruses. They usually detect a potential pathogen by 'recognising' an unfamiliar protein or sugar on its surface. This protein or sugar is called an *antigen*. B-cells then divide rapidly and produce daughter cells whose task it is to manufacture antibodies to the antigen. These daughter cells carry out their work at a phenomenal rate, manufacturing many antibodies every second. Some of them also act as memory cells, retaining a memory of the antigen so that more antibody can be produced if it is needed in the future.

Antibodies work in a variety of ways depending on the kind of micro-organism they encounter. Some of them give the pathogen a special covering which makes it easier for phagocytes to engulf it. Others neutralise the poisonous substances or toxins produced by pathogens. Some antibodies may actually destroy virus particles or prevent them from binding to cells (Figure 7).

Figure 7: Processes involving B-cells

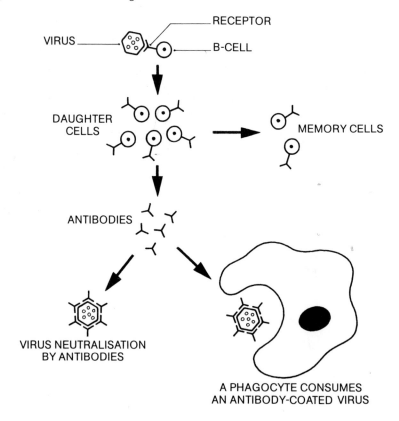

B-cells are, however, unable to cope in circumstances where a micro-organism has already entered a host cell and has begun to reproduce itself. Whilst they can produce antibodies to contain the pathogen outside the host cell, they can do little to affect the process by which the pathogen reproduces itself within it. T-cells, on the other hand, can deal with such a situation.

T-cells   There are thousands of different kinds of T-cells but they can all be divided into four basic types:

Killer or Cytotoxic T-cells
Helper T-cells
Suppressor T-cells
Memory T-cells

Killer or Cytotoxic T-cells have the ability to destroy other cells in the body that have been infected by viruses or bacteria. Suppressor T-cells help damp down the activity of the immune system after Killer T-cells have been at work. Memory T-cells act, as their name suggests, by 'remembering' the kind of infection that has been dealt with. They 'switch on' the relevant part of the immune system quickly the next time a similar pathogen is encountered.

Helper T-cells, however, are those that have the most crucial role in regulating the activity of the immune system. They co-ordinate the actions of phagocytes, encourage B-cells to produce antibodies and stimulate Killer T-cells to deal with virus- or bacteria-infected cells. If they are lost in significant numbers or if their function becomes disturbed, problems can ensue.

While T-cells can not be told apart when looked at under the microscope, they can be distinguished by the different chemical markers they have on their outer surfaces. Some of these markers are common to all T-cells but others are more specific. Two of these markers are particularly important within the context of HIV infection and AIDS. These are the T4 marker (or CD4 marker as it is sometimes called) which is present on the surface of Helper T-cells, and the T8 (or CD8) marker which is present on the surface of Suppressor T-cells (Figure 8).

Figure 8: Processes involving T-cells

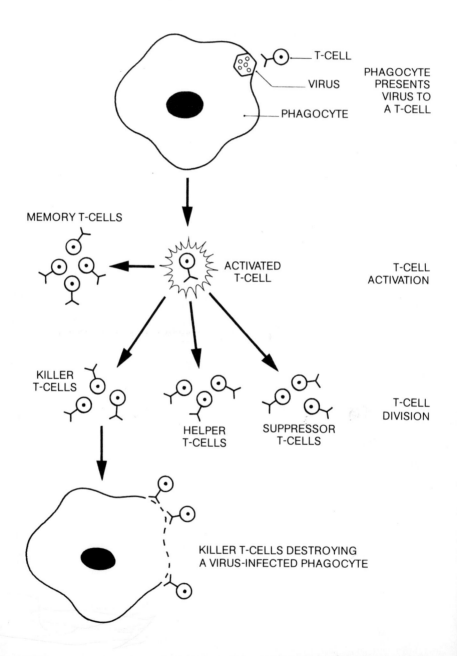

AIDS and the immune system

For some time before HIV was identified, certain well-documented changes were known to take place in the immune system just before or at the same time as a person developed AIDS. The most significant of these was a change in the proportion of T-cells carrying the T4 surface marker. In most healthy people, about 60% of T-cells carry the T4 surface marker (Helper T-cells) and about 30% carry the T8 marker (Suppressor T-cells). This means that when a person is healthy, their Helper/Suppressor ratio will be about 2:1. In people diagnosed with AIDS, however, this ratio is generally much lower and may even be reversed. Subsequently, it has been shown that this change in the ratio of Helper T-cells to Suppressor T-cells is brought about by a decrease in the number of Helper T-cells. It is now known that HIV has a strong affinity for the T4 surface receptor on Helper T-cells and that it gains entry to the cell through these receptors. Thereafter it may remain dormant for months, even years.

Scientists are still unclear about the factors that cause HIV to reproduce itself, but once this starts to happen, T-cells are destroyed, producing the altered ratio of Helper T-cells to Suppressor T-cells. Changes may also take place in those Helper T-cells that are not infected or which survive viral replication. Many of these seem unable to recognise antigens previously encountered and are unable to organise an effective response to subsequent infection. HIV may have an effect on B-cells too, stimulating them to produce high levels of HIV antibody, thereby 'distracting' them from the work that they need to carry out in order to deal effectively with other pathogens.

Other cells in the body apart from Helper T-cells also have the T4 surface marker. In particular, some cells in the brain carry it and HIV has now been isolated from brain tissue. It has been suggested that some of the psychological disturbances associated with HIV encephalopathy may be a direct consequence of the virus's effects on brain tissue.

1.4   VIRUSES

Because a particular virus has now been identified in connection with AIDS, it is important to recognise in general terms what viruses are, what they do and how they reproduce themselves.

Viruses are the simplest living organisms known. They consist of a core of genetic material in the form of Deoxyribonucleic acid (DNA) or Ribonucleic acid (RNA) surrounded by a coat of protein. This, in turn is surrounded by another protective layer or envelope (Figure 9).

Figure 9: The main features of a virus

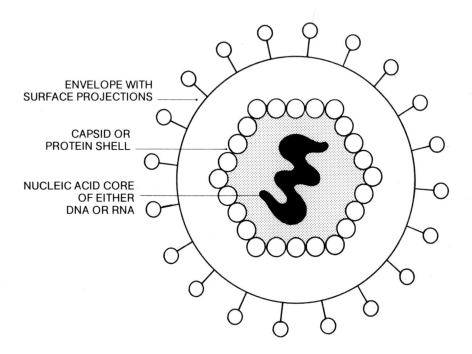

ENVELOPE WITH
SURFACE PROJECTIONS

CAPSID OR
PROTEIN SHELL

NUCLEIC ACID CORE
OF EITHER
DNA OR RNA

In order for a virus to reproduce, its genetic material must get inside a cell. Once this has happened, it can then influence the functions of the cell so that more virus can be produced. This process takes place in a number of steps. First, proteins on the outer surface (or envelope) of the virus 'latch' themselves onto receptor proteins on the surface of cells to which the virus has an affinity. Then, the inner core of the virus containing genetic material is 'injected' into the body cell. This inner core, which is usually made up of the chemical DNA, then finds its way to the nucleus of the body cell where it 'hijacks' the host cell's normal metabolic processes so that the cell becomes a 'factory' for the production of more virus. In order for this to occur, the virus's own DNA has to become integrated into the DNA of the host cell. The genes of the virus and the genes of the host cell become one and the same (Figure 10).

Figure 10: The life cycle of a virus

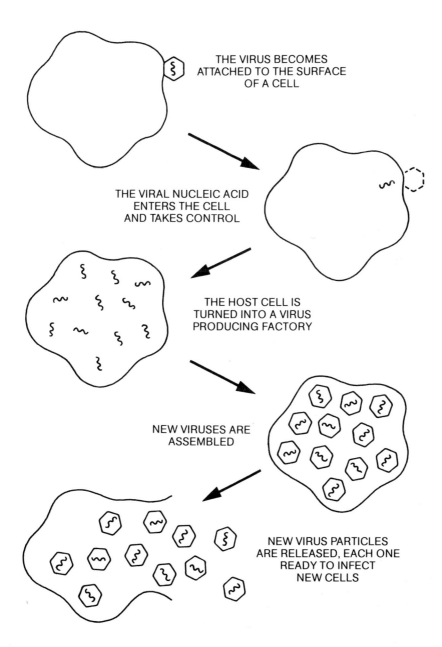

Why are viruses described as living things?

To describe a virus as a living thing is not to imply that it has thoughts, feelings and intentions, although everyday speech and the language of certain textbooks might suggest that this is the case. We sometimes read, for example, of viruses 'being attracted' to certain kinds of cells, of them 'having a preference' for a certain host or of them 'attacking' a particular species. This kind of language, which gives viruses human qualities, can of course be very misleading because it implies that they 'choose' when, where, how and who they will infect. It may also encourage some people to feel that they are not at risk of infection because they do not fall into a group which a particular virus supposedly 'prefers'. For example, because in Europe and North America, HIV infection was first identified in gay men, and because as yet there have been fewer reported cases of heterosexual transmission in these parts of the world, some heterosexual people in the West may imagine that they are not at risk of infection when they have unprotected sex. In reality, provided the conditions for transmission are appropriate, viruses are quite unselective in whom they infect.

Retroviruses

The genetic blueprint of most viruses is stored in the form of the chemical DNA. A few viruses differ from this, however, since their genetic material is stored in the form of a related but different chemical called RNA. These viruses are called *retroviruses*.

Until relatively recently, retroviruses were better known to vets than to doctors since they were known to cause certain kinds of cancers as well as immune deficiency in animals. Feline leukaemia virus, for example, is a retrovirus that causes an acquired immune deficiency in cats, and visna is a retrovirus that causes a similar condition in sheep. Animals with visna frequently develop pneumonia, but infection by this retrovirus is also associated with progressive degeneration of nervous tissue, particularly the brain.

The first human retroviruses were identified in the 1970s. The first to be detected was the virus responsible for human T-cell leukaemia. It is called Human T-cell Lymphotropic Virus Type 1 (HTLV-I). Soon afterwards a closely related but much rarer human leukaemia virus was identified which was named HTLV-II.

Retroviruses differ from the majority of viruses in that their genetic material is stored in the form of a chemical called RNA rather than in DNA. In order for their genetic material to become integrated into that of the host cell, which itself consists of DNA, retroviral RNA must first be changed into DNA. This is accomplished via a special enzyme contained within the retrovirus called *reverse transcriptase.* The DNA which contains a blueprint for the production of more virus can then be integrated into the host cell's own DNA (Figure 11).

Figure 11: The life cycle of a retrovirus

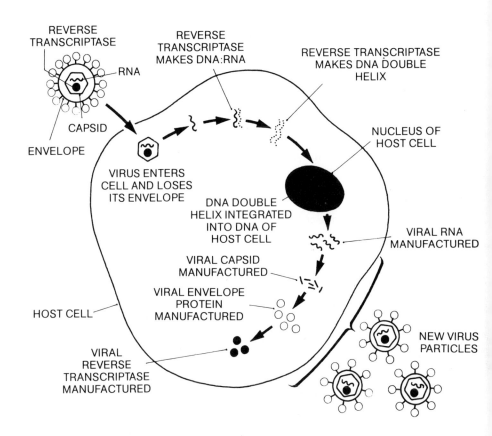

Human Immunodeficiency Virus

For some time before HIV was first isolated, it had been suspected that AIDS might be caused by a human retrovirus. Several pieces of evidence suggested this. First, as we have seen it was known that a variety of acquired immune deficiency states in animals were caused by retroviruses. Second, AIDS was known to be associated with T-cell abnormalities, and two retroviruses had already been isolated which infected T-cells (HTLV-I and HTLV-II). Third, it was sometimes possible to observe reverse transcriptase activity in T-cell cultures obtained from people with AIDS.

In 1983, a team led by Luc Montagnier of the Pasteur Institute in Paris, announced that they had isolated a retrovirus from the swollen lymph nodes of a person with Lymphadenopathy Syndrome (Barre-Sinoussi *et al*, 1984). They called this virus Lymphadenopathy Virus (LAV). About a year afterwards, researchers in Robert Gallo's laboratory at the National Cancer Institute in the United States reported that they too had isolated a retrovirus, this time from people with AIDS. They called their virus Human T-Cell Lymphotropic Virus Type III (HTLV-III). Subsequently, a third team led by Jay Levy at the University of California, San Francisco also announced they had isolated a retrovirus from people with AIDS. They called this virus AIDS-Associated Retrovirus (ARV) (Levy *et al*, 1984).

These viruses have been shown to be genetically similar, but not identical, to one another, and whilst the old nomenclature continues to be used occasionally, they are now known collectively as Human Immunodeficiency Virus (HIV). In terms of its structure we now know that HIV is very similar to other retroviruses. It has an RNA core which is surrounded by two layers of protein (named p24 and p18) and an outer fatty membrane or envelope. This envelope has a number of proteins with sugars, *glycoproteins*, embedded in it (Figure 12).

Figure 12: The structure of HIV

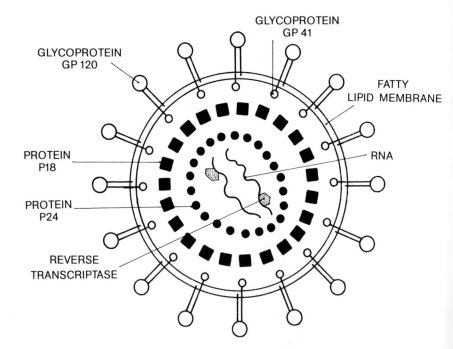

Within a remarkably short period of time, the genetic structure of HIV has been worked out. A great deal is now known about the genes that make up the virus. Four of these are of particular importance: the *gag* gene which codes the proteins that make up the core of the virus, the *pol* gene which codes for the production of the enzyme reverse transcriptase which is needed for viral replication, the *env* gene which codes for the protein envelope that surrounds the viral core, and the *tat-III* gene (sometimes known as the *trans* activator gene) which switches on viral replication. Without the *tat-III* gene, HIV is unable to reproduce itself.

While certain aspects of the genetic structure of HIV remain constant across different strains of the virus, others differ. In particular, it is now known that there is considerable variability in the portion of viral RNA that relates to the protein envelope that surrounds the genetic core of the virus. This variability occurs both in samples of the virus obtained from different people (there are marked differences between samples obtained on the West Coast of America and samples obtained on the East Coast, for example) and in samples obtained from the same person at different points in time. This suggests that there is a high rate of spontaneous change in the genetic material that relates to this part of the virus. More recently, a Human Immunodeficiency Virus which differs markedly in its genetic structure from any of the samples previously obtained has been identified among people resident in West Africa, Portugal, Brazil and France. This virus has been named HIV-II to distinguish it from earlier isolates. It is much rarer than HIV (which in some quarters has now been re-named HIV-I) and early evidence suggests that it is likely to have similar effects on the human immune system.

1.5 THERAPY

Being diagnosed as HIV positive or as having AIDS is generally an extremely frightening experience. In the former situation, there may be uncertainty concerning the eventual outcome of the diagnosis. In the latter, there may be anxiety about the likely progression of the syndrome. In both of these situations, there will be a need for high-quality care, and choices may have to be made between the various options on offer. Once they have accepted their initial diagnosis, individuals may feel bewildered by the range of alternative therapies open to them. It is therefore important to receive the best possible advice at this critical time.

Help for people with HIV infection or AIDS can increasingly be obtained in both the statutory and voluntary sectors. Some support may be provided through STD Clinics and Departments of Genito-Urinary Medicine where many cases of HIV infection are first identified. A number of these units now work in close co-operation with voluntary sector organisations providing services for people affected by HIV infection. GPs also have an important role to play in meeting the needs of those with HIV infection and AIDS. In recent years, the growing tendency towards community-based medicine has encouraged some doctors to explore the advantages of a more holistic approach to care, viewing illness not as an isolated phenomenon but within the broader context of an individual's life and the society of which she or he is a part.

There are also options to be considered within the field of alternative and complementary medicine. Health care of this kind may be controversial, but there are many people with HIV infection or AIDS who claim to have benefited from it. It will ultimately be for the individual to decide on the most appropriate kind of therapy, but help in reaching a decision may come from voluntary sector organisations with a knowledge of local facilities. In London for example, Frontliners, a group of people with AIDS, have carried out a borough-by-borough survey of the city's services, and Body Positive groups around the country have accumulated a wealth of information about different approaches to health care, both physical and psychological. Advice on the value of different kinds of therapies is now available in a number of publications (Callen & Herman, 1987; Frontliners, 1987).

Drugs

There are a number of drugs that are effective against the opportunistic diseases associated with AIDS. PCP, for example, can be treated effectively with either co-trimoxazole (Septrin) or pentamidine and, provided therapy begins early enough, most people will recover from at least their first bout of infection. A combination of sulphadiazine and pyrimethamine is usually used to treat toxoplasmosis, and here too the response is usually good so long as treatment is started early. Fungal infections such as candida can be treated either topically by clotrimazole or nystatin, or systemically by ketoconazole. Viral infections such as herpes can now be successfully managed with acyclovir, and cytomegaloviral infection responds reasonably well to treatment with a new drug ganciclovir. Efforts have also been made to treat KS using radiotherapy and chemotherapy as well as with α-interferon. The various treatments available for opportunistic diseases associated with AIDS have been discussed at length by Weller (1987) and Young (1987).

Unfortunately, many of these drugs need to be administered in large doses if treatment is to be successful, and this means that side effects often occur. Sometimes these may be so severe as to require the discontinuation of therapy, but more often they mean that opportunistic diseases cannot be treated as aggressively as physicians might otherwise wish. Nevertheless, provided treatment begins early enough, the quality of life open to people with AIDS can be significantly improved.

While a number of drugs are effective against the opportunistic diseases associated with AIDS, few can be used to treat HIV infection itself or the immune deficiency it causes. Being a retrovirus, HIV also poses special problems so far as drug therapy is concerned because in order to replicate it has to integrate itself into the host's own genetic makeup. Therefore, drugs designed to deal with the virus may also affect vital host cells.

The ideal antiviral drug will have to do several things. First, it will have to stop viral production in cells that have already been infected. Second, it will have to have a regenerative effect on the immune system. Third, in view of what we now know about HIV encephalopathy, it will have to be capable of crossing the blood/brain barrier. Finally, it must have few side effects because it will have to be taken for life. Identifying a single drug which has all of these qualities is clearly a difficult task, and researchers are now more confident that the desired results can be achieved with a combination of therapies.

There are now a number of drugs that can slow down or stop HIV production in an infected person. The best known of these is zidovudine (AZT or Retrovir) which works by interfering with the enzyme reverse transcriptase which HIV needs in order to replicate. Zidovudine has been shown to reduce significantly mortality and morbidity amongst people with AIDS. It is also effective in the treatment of ARC, and there have been preliminary reports that it can reverse some of the damage associated with HIV encephalopathy (Yenchoan et al, 1987). It does, however, have a number of side effects which include bone marrow damage, anaemia, nausea, insomnia and muscular pains. People receiving the drug may be in need of frequent blood transfusions in order to compensate for some of these problems.

A number of other drugs are currently undergoing clinical trials. These include dideoxycytidine which, in combination with zidovudine, seems to give promising results (Yarchoan, 1988), ampligen, ribavirin, castanospermine and fusidic acid. A number of other drugs have been tested in the laboratory for their *in vitro* effects upon HIV. Clinical trials involving some of them can be expected in the near future.

There has been considerable controversy about the effectiveness of an egg lecithin product called AL 721 as a treatment for HIV infection and AIDS. Double blind control trials have shown that one of its ingredients (phosphatidylcholine) may be effective against certain kinds of viral infection, and reports from a number of ongoing studies of people with AIDS taking AL 721 suggest that there may be subjective benefit to be gained from this kind of therapy (James, 1987). Doctors in Britain, however, remain divided about its use.

Vaccines

Until recently, scientists have felt that it would be extremely difficult to produce an effective vaccine against HIV infection. In part, this was believed to be so because of HIV's genetic variability. There are many slightly different strains of HIV, and even within the same individual, the virus seems to mutate and change its structure over time. This poses major problems for vaccine development.

It is now clear that, in spite of this variability, certain features of HIV remain relatively constant. In particular, it is now known that certain parts of the virus's glycoprotein coat (gp 120) remain constant across all strains, allowing it to bind to the T4 receptors that can be found on certain types of cells. Various kinds of trial vaccines are currently being synthesised using this knowledge. Some of them combine this element of the virus's coat with an immune-stimulating complex, an iscom, which encourages the production of neutralising antibodies to this part of the virus.

Other approaches to vaccine development involve the insertion of non-harmful HIV genes, such as those coding for its coat, into other 'carrier' viruses. As part of the body's natural response to these 'carrier' viruses, it is anticipated that neutralising antibodies to parts of HIV itself will be produced. Trials of vaccines developed in this way are now taking place.

There may be problems, however, with both of these approaches since they assume that the body can mount an effective antibody response against HIV. Given that the antibodies produced to HIV infection tend to be unable to neutralise the virus, and given that they fail to prevent the progression of disease in many people, we can only be cautiously optimistic about the outcomes of these studies. Vaccine development is clearly in its infancy, and even assuming that some of the studies now underway prove successful, it is unlikely that a vaccine will be available before the early 1990s.

Holistic therapy

Whilst clinical medicine has proved increasingly effective in treating some of the opportunistic infections associated with AIDS, as yet it can do little to strengthen the damaged immune system itself. In consequence, a number of people with HIV infection and AIDS have turned to alternative and complementary medicine as a way of challenging the general fatalism that surrounds AIDS. As Tatchell (1986) has put it,

'. . . People who are infected with the virus are not powerless and helpless. Instead of accepting their fate as passive victims who re-define themselves as patients and slide irreversibly into the "sick role", people with HIV infection and AIDS can make the conscious, positive choice to mentally and physically fight the disease. . . .'

There are many different kinds of holistic therapy available for people with HIV infection or AIDS. These range from acupuncture, acupressure, homoeopathy, hypnotherapy and spiritual healing to meditation, yoga, visualisation and relaxation training. All suggest that attention should be given to diet, exercise and rest, and psychological and emotional well-being, if the body's capacity for self-healing is to be maximised.

A sound diet is always important as the basis for good health, and advice from a professional nutritionist may be sought on this. Much has been written about the possible enhancement of the immune system by vitamin or mineral supplements, but as Gay Men's Health Crisis, the New York-based self-help organisation for people with AIDS, has recently pointed out, many exaggerated claims have been made for the effectiveness of these kinds of intervention (GMHC, 1987). The most important thing to aim for is a balanced diet to provide the immune system with the support it needs.

It is important for people with HIV infection to get adequate sleep and exercise. Rest may be particularly essential since there may not only be the stress of the medical diagnosis to live with but the ignorance and prejudice of others. Reasonable levels of exercise may also reinforce self-esteem and confidence as well as physical strength. It is therefore important that people with HIV infection are offered the opportunity to share their feelings with others in order to work through damaging emotional reactions and in order to enhance self-esteem. Different kinds of relaxation therapy may be useful in this area.

References

Barre-Sinoussi, F. *et al* (1984) Isolation of a T-lymphotropic retrovirus from a patient at risk for AIDS, *Science,* **220,** p 868.

Beldekas J. *et al* (1986) African Swine Fever and AIDS, *Lancet,* **i,** pp 564–5.

Callen, M. & Herman, B. (1987) What to look for in a doctor, in *Surviving and Thriving with AIDS,* New York, People with AIDS Coalition Inc.

CDC (1987) CDC Revised Case-definition for AIDS, in M. Youle *et al AIDS: Therapeutics in HIV Disease,* London, Churchill Livingstone.

Ciraru-Vigneron, N. *et al* (1987) HIV infection among high risk pregnant women, *Lancet,* **i,** p 630.

Duesberg, P. H. (1987) Retroviruses as carcinogens and pathogens: expectations and realities, *Cancer Research,* 47, pp 1199–1220.

Eales, L. *et al* (1987) Association of different allelic forms of group specific component with susceptibility to and clinical manifestations of HIV infection, *Lancet,* **i,** pp 999–1002.

Eales, L. *et al* (1988) Group specific component and AIDS: erroneous data, *Lancet,* **i,** p 936.

Frontliners (1987) *Living with AIDS,* London, Frontliners.

GMHC (1987) Nutrition and AIDS, *Treatment Issues,* **i,** 1.

James, J. (1987) AL 721 Today, *New York Native,* **243,** pp 17–18.

Lauritsen, J. (1986) *Death rush – poppers and AIDS,* New York, Pagan Press.

Levy, J. *et al* (1984) Isolation of lympathocytopathic retroviruses from San Francisco patients with AIDS, in R. Kulstad (ed.) *AIDS: Papers from Science.* Washington, American Association for the Advancement of Science.

Lo, S. (1986) Isolation and identification of a novel virus from patients with AIDS, *American Journal of Tropical Medicine and Hygiene,* **35** 4, pp 675–6.

Nixon, D. *et al* (1987) Group specific component and HIV infection, *Lancet,* **ii,** pp 40–1.

Pinching, A. & Jefferies, D. (1985) AIDS and HTLV-III/LAV infection: consequences for obstetrics and perinatal medicine, *British Journal of Obstetrics and Gynaecology,* **92,** pp 1211–17.

Tatchell, P. (1986) *AIDS: A Guide to Survival,* London, Gay Men's Press.

Weber, J. *et al* (1986) Factors affecting seropositivity for HTLV-III/LAV and progression of the disease in partners of patients with AIDS, *Lancet,* **i,** pp 1179–81.

Weller, I. (1987) Treatment of infections and antiviral agents, *British Medical Journal,* **295,** pp 200–204.

WHO (1988) Statistics made available at the World Summit of Health Ministers, London.

Yarchoan, R. *et al* (1988) Phase 1 studies of 2′ 3′ Dideoxycytidine in severe HIV infection as a single agent and alternatively with zidovudine, *Lancet,* **i,** p 76–80.

Yenchoan, R. *et al* (1987) Response of Human Immunodeficiency Virus associated neurological disease to 3′-azido-3′-deoxythymidine, *Lancet,* **i,** pp 132–5.

Young, L. (1987) Treatable aspects of infection due to Human Immunodeficiency Virus, *Lancet,* **ii,** pp 1503–6.

2.   Epidemiology and transmission

2.1   WHAT IS EPIDEMIOLOGY?

Epidemiology is the study of the distribution and determinants of disease within and between different groups of people. It aims to identify the frequency with which particular diseases occur as well as the characteristics of those who are affected (Barker & Rose, 1984). Of particular interest to epidemiologists are changing patterns of disease since these can reveal much about the growth and decline of epidemics. Findings from epidemiological research can be used to identify changing health care needs within the community. They can also inform the development of health and social policy.

Major sources of data used by epidemiologists are mortality and morbidity statistics. The former are obtained from death certificates, whereas the latter are obtained from hospital records, general practitioners and the official notification of certain infectious diseases. Occasionally, epidemiologists carry out surveys to identify the prevalence of diseases within particular populations, as well as the incidence of new cases. The conclusions reached by epidemiologists are therefore critically dependent on the quality and accuracy of the data collected. For a variety of reasons, morbidity statistics (and to a lesser extent mortality statistics) may be incomplete or inaccurate. Care should therefore be taken in the interpretation of epidemiological findings (Prior, 1985; Bloor *et al.*, 1987).

2.2   RISK FACTORS

Of particular interest to epidemiologists are the *risk factors* associated with particular diseases, since these can form the basis for preventative measures. In the case of a new or newly recognised condition, there can be special difficulties in identifying risk factors, since it may be necessary to work backwards from the signs and symptoms that can presently be observed to identify earlier stages in the natural history of the disease. In retrospective studies like this, large numbers of shared behavioural traits and patterns may be observed and the difficulty lies in determining which of these are the most significant. However, by comparing members of a given social group who have the disease with others from the same group without it, it is possible to isolate the significant risk factors that might form the basis for preventative measures. This technique is known as a *case-control study*.

In their efforts to identify risk factors, epidemiologists also compare people who have been exposed to the suspected causal agent with those who have not.

This technique is known as a *cohort study*. In this way, the average length of time between infection and the appearance of symptoms can be established, together with an indication of the groups that are most at risk. These are often referred to as high-risk groups.

2.3 HIGH-RISK GROUPS

Using the techniques identified above, and before HIV was isolated, epidemiologists were able to identify a number of risk factors for AIDS. Some of these were of a general nature, such as being Haitian, being a gay man or being an injecting drug user. Others were more specific and identified particular behaviours or particular acts. These included the number of sexual partners an individual had, the recreational use of nitrite inhalants, and anal sex, particularly receptive anal sex. As a consequence of this, from early on in the epidemic, Haitians, gay and bisexual men, injecting drug users, prostitutes and the 'promiscuous' came to be understood as high-risk groups. They were subsequently joined by haemophiliacs and the recipients of blood transfusions.

It is important to recognise that the nature of risk factors may change over time in response to health education. Thus, the adoption of safer drug-related practices may have significantly altered the extent to which injecting drug use is still a risk factor. For those who inject but never share equipment, injection is no longer a risk factor, whereas for those who still share syringes and needles, it has remained so. Distinctions such as these should encourage health educators to differentiate between *possible* risk factors and the *actual* mechanisms by which disease is transmitted. This distinction is vitally important in contemporary discussion about the number of sexual partners a person has.

The number of sexual partners that someone has will undoubtedly increase the statistical likelihood of them coming into contact (in the sense of meeting) with a person who is already infected. In the early days of the epidemic, when little was known about the cause of AIDS, the number of sexual partners did indeed play a significant role in predicting in case-control studies those who were most likely to develop AIDS. However, subsequent knowledge about HIV's modes of transmission has dramatically changed this situation, and it is important to realise that this potential risk will remain insignificant so long as the sexual behaviour of the individuals concerned does not allow HIV to be transmitted. Thus, if safer sex guidelines are strictly followed with every partner (see Chapter 6) and no exchange of semen, blood, vaginal or cervical secretions takes place, then having more than one sexual partner will *not* in itself increase the risk of transmission. Only if there is an exchange of these fluids will this risk be increased.

It is therefore vitally important for health educators to distinguish between the ways in which HIV is transmitted in *individuals' everyday lives,* and theoretical risk factors that may apply, or may have applied in the past to abstract *general populations*. The confusion between these two levels of analysis has led to much controversy concerning who actually is at risk of HIV (Adler, 1987).

In many ways, the statistical concept of high- and low-risk groups, as opposed to high- and low-risk activities, has tended to obscure rather than to clarify understanding of the risks that confront individuals. As an unintended consequence, it may also have encouraged complacency amongst those who have been led to picture themselves in apparently 'safe' categories.

2.4 THE EPIDEMIOLOGY OF HIV INFECTION AND AIDS

While the first reported cases of AIDS occurred in the United States in 1981 following the diagnosis of Pneumocystis carinii pneumonia and Kaposi's sarcoma in gay men, subsequent retrospective studies have shown that there were cases of AIDS in Europe, America and Africa in the late 1970s. The cause of the syndrome and its modes of transmission were not immediately apparent, however, and it was not until late 1983 that HIV was identified.

Subsequently, the development of antibody and antigen tests has enabled sophisticated epidemiological studies of the epidemic to be carried out in many parts of the world. Care should be taken, however, in interpreting the results of these studies since political considerations, social taboos and other factors have contributed to an under-reporting of cases of HIV infection in some countries. Moreover, in some parts of the world, AIDS itself has been under-recognised and under-diagnosed. In consequence, reported cases of HIV infection and AIDS may not represent the true prevalence of disease (WHO, 1987).

It is important to distinguish between the epidemiology of HIV and the epidemiology of AIDS. AIDS statistics are usually obtained from morbidity and mortality records. Estimates of the prevalence and incidence of HIV infection, however, are less reliable since they are likely to be based either on findings from cohort studies or from the notification of voluntary HIV antibody tests which cannot be taken as representative or exhaustive. Because of this unreliability, there have been, and continue to be, strong demands for routine but anonymous HIV screening (see Chapter 3 for a fuller discussion of these issues). As the World Health Organization (WHO) has pointed out, 'Accurate AIDS data is critical as the base to assess the future impact of AIDS on health care systems, national economies and demographic patterns' (WHO, 1987). This kind of information is also of importance to health educators evaluating the effectiveness of different kinds of intervention.

The global picture

AIDS By December 1988, a total of 132,976 cases of AIDS from 152 different countries had been reported to WHO. Due to delays and difficulties in reporting, however, the real number of cases is currently estimated to be over 200,000. Over 70% of these are in North and South America (mostly in the United States), 13%

in Europe, and 16% in African countries. In Africa and the Caribbean, men and women are affected in equal numbers. Globally, 75%-90% of AIDS cases presently occur among people aged 20-40, and in the hardest-hit African cities, death rates among babies and young adults can be expected to increase rapidly. In this kind of situation, HIV does not have to spread rapidly to have a significant cumulative effect, and as the director of the WHO AIDS Programme has recently put it, 'We are still in the early phases of a global epidemic whose first decade gives every reason for concern about the future' (Mann, 1988)

HIV infection   There are no reliable statistics concerning the global incidence of HIV infection, but WHO estimated in early 1988 that between five and ten million persons may be currently infected. By 1991, WHO calculates that at least one million new cases of AIDS could develop in people already infected, the results from recent epidemiological cohort-study research suggesting that 'we should regard progression to clinical AIDS after infection with HIV as the norm rather than the exception' (Moss, 1988).

The United States
AIDS   In the United States, where the most detailed epidemiological research has taken place, 80,538 cases of AIDS had been reported by December 1988. This figure makes up almost two thirds of all reported cases worldwide. Of these cases, about half have already died, and by 1991, the Centers for Disease Control (CDC) currently estimates the cumulative total of cases will reach 270,000, of whom 179,000 will be dead. The vast majority of cases in the United States are adults and adolescents, with paediatric cases currently accounting for less than 2% of the total. By age, two thirds of those affected are in the 20-39 year group and almost 90% in the 20-49 year group. By sex, 90% of adult and adolescent cases are males. By risk group, 69% of the adult and adolescent cases are gay or bisexual males, including 7% who are also injecting drug users. Heterosexual injecting drug users make up the other major group of people with AIDS, accounting for 20% of the cumulative total. Of the remainder, 4% have been infected by heterosexual contact and 4% are haemophiliacs or other persons who have received infected blood transfusions or blood products.

   By race and ethnicity, minorities make up a disproportionate number of people with AIDS in the United States. Blacks make up 27% of all AIDS cases, yet comprise only 12% of the total population. Hispanics make up 13% of AIDS cases, yet are 6% of the total population and 59% of AIDS cases are among whites who make up 80% of the total population. Looking at risk groups by race and ethnicity, 73% of gay and bisexual males with AIDS are white, while 80% of injecting drug users with AIDS are black or Hispanic. Of children with AIDS, 78% are the children of parents at risk. The vast majority of these children are black or Hispanic. AIDS is already the leading cause of death in New York among men aged 25-44, and women aged 25-34.

HIV infection   Estimates of the number of people with HIV infection in the United States vary considerably from a low of 276,000 to a high of 1,750,000. A number of cohort studies have enabled estimates to be made of the proportion of different groups affected. These estimates vary considerably, however, depending on the cohort studied: a finding which raises questions about the value of identifying risk groups rather than risk behaviours (see Section 2.3). Depending on the study cited, between 24–68% of gay and bisexual men may be infected, between 2–72% of injecting drug users, between 0–40% of prostitutes and between 40–79% of haemophiliacs.

In making sense of findings like these, it is important to remember that many of those affected acquired HIV infection before the virus itself had been identified and before its modes of transmission were understood. Infection spread rapidly in this context, infecting half or more of the gay men surveyed in cities like New York, San Francisco, Philadelphia and Denver. There is now considerable evidence that the rate of new infection amongst this group at least has declined dramatically and in one cohort study based in San Francisco, the rate of new infections per year peaked at 21% of the group in 1982 but fell to a single new infection in 1986 and in 1987 (Boffey, 1988).

The United Kingdom
In England, Wales and Northern Ireland, cases of AIDS and deaths from the syndrome are reported in confidence to the Communicable Disease Surveillance Centre (CDSC). In Scotland, figures are reported separately to the Communicable Diseases (Scotland) Unit. The accuracy of reporting is increased by co-operation with the Office of Population, Censuses and Surveys (OPCS), which also sends in confidence copies of death certificates mentioning AIDS to both of these organisations. The most readily available source of information concerning the epidemiology of HIV and AIDS in the United Kingdom are the quarterly figures published by the Department of Health. The Health Education Authority in London also publishes a quarterly epidemiological briefing on AIDS/HIV in the United Kingdom, entitled *AIDS-UK.*

AIDS By the end of June 1989, the cumulative total figure of people with AIDS in the UK was 2,372, of whom 1,272 had died (Figure 13). For Britain as a whole, 81% of reported cases of AIDS were gay or bisexual men, 6% were haemophiliacs and 4% were women (PHLS, 1989) Approximately 70% of AIDS cases were diagnosed in people aged 25-44, and another 20% in people aged 45-64.

Figure 13: UK AIDS cases by patient characteristic:
Cumulative total to end of June 1989

	Males	Females	Total	Deaths
Homosexual/Bisexual	1,927	0	1,927	1,023
Injecting drug users	44	17	61	28
Homosexual male and injecting drug users	33	–	33	15
Haemophiliac	147	2	149	93
Recipient of blood				
Abroad	10	14	24	15
UK	12	5	17	14
Heterosexual				
Possibly infected				
Abroad	52	24	76	37
UK	11	15	26	14
· Child at risk/infected parent	9	13	22	11
Undetermined	32	5	37	22
TOTALS	2,277	95	2,372	1,272

(Prepared by CDSC and CD [Scotland] Unit)

These figures do not allow for possible under-reporting, and in some circumstances AIDS may not be mentioned on a death certificate in order to spare relatives from possible embarrassment. Some GPs may also be unaware of the extent of the AIDS epidemic, so there is still the possibility that patients dying from HIV-related conditions may not have been diagnosed as such (Boyton & Scambler, 1988). The CDSC has recently been reported as suggesting that perhaps twice as many people may have died from AIDS as are stated in official figures (McCormick, 1988). More accurate reporting can be expected as knowledge about HIV and AIDS increases among doctors and the general public.

HIV infection By the end of June 1989, there were 10,794 reported cases of HIV infection in the UK (HEA, 1989). Of these, 8,934 were in England, 131 in Wales, 1,688 in Scotland, 61 in Northern Ireland. 48% of the individuals were gay or bisexual men, 16% injecting drug users, 11% the recipients of infected blood or blood products, including haemophiliacs, 6% infected through heterosexual contact, and 18% of undetermined exposure category. The Thames Health Regions accounted for 57% of reported cases, the rest of England 26%, Scotland 15% and Wales and Northern Ireland 2%. Overall, about 87% of those affected were men, and the majority were aged between 20-29. Whilst gay and bisexual men made up the majority of reported cases in London, injecting drug users predominated in Scotland, and the recipients of infected blood or blood products made up the majority of those affected in the rest of England, Wales and Northern Ireland.

It is important to recognise that regional variations in the reported incidence of HIV infection should not be regarded as an accurate index of the prevalence of infection in different parts of the country. For a variety of reasons, people may attend for a test in a region other than that in which they live, and laboratories reporting a positive result may be in a different region to that in which the test was carried out (DHSS, 1988).

2.5 TRANSMISSION

Given the confusion that presently exists about the ways in which HIV is and is not transmitted, it is important in health education to differentiate between the body fluids and tissues from which HIV has been *isolated* and the body fluids and tissues through which it is *transmitted.*

HIV has now been isolated from many body fluids and tissues including,

blood	semen
vaginal and cervical secretions	breast milk
saliva	tears
amniotic fluid	cerebro-spinal fluid
most body organs	skin

However, simply because a micro-organism can be isolated from a particular tissue or fluid does not mean that it is necessarily transmitted in that way. For example, many potentially lethal micro-organisms can be cultivated under sophisticated laboratory conditions from smears taken from table tops, work surfaces or other objects that people regularly come into contact with. This does not mean that these micro-organisms are necessarily transmitted via these surfaces. For transmission to take place, a critical quantity of a micro-organism (an inoculum) must pass from one person to another via a critical route specific to that micro-organism (see Section 1.3).

Much of what we presently understand about the ways in which HIV is and is not transmitted comes from three different kinds of research: epidemiological studies looking at the groups most affected by HIV infection, sexual contact studies and studies of households, hospitals and workplaces.

How HIV is transmitted

Transmission studies show quite unequivocally that HIV can be transmitted via the following fluids and tissues:

semen	blood products
vaginal and cervical secretions	organ transplants
blood	

Sexual transmission   The virus can be transmitted from man to man (Kingsley *et al*, 1987), from man to woman (Calabrese & Gopalakrishna, 1986), and from woman to man (Fischi *et al*, 1987) through penetrative sex without a condom. HIV has also been transmitted via artificial insemination by donor (Stewart *et al*, 1985), although HIV antibody tests are now carried out on donors to ensure that the risks associated with this procedure are minimal. There is also some evidence that sexual transmission from woman to woman can take place (Marmor *et al*, 1986; Monzon and Capellan, 1987).

Among gay men, anal sex without a condom is the activity which carries the greatest risk, particularly to the receptive partner (Kingsley *et al*, 1987), and anal sex between a woman and a man may carry a similar risk. It is now clear that in some cases transmission takes place with the first sexual contact whereas in others even repeated sexual contact may not result in infection.

A detailed discussion of many of the issues involved in sexual transmission can be found in Chapters 5 and 6.

Transmission via blood and blood products   HIV can be transmitted whenever an exchange of blood takes place between two people. This has occurred via blood transfusions, via infected blood products and via the sharing of syringes and hypodermic needles.

HIV transmission via blood transfusions was first recognised in 1983 (Amman *et al*, 1983; Esteban *et al*, 1985), and since September 1985, all donated blood in Britain has been screened for antibodies to HIV, and any infected blood has been rejected.

The antibody testing of donated blood is generally extremely effective, although there is a very slight possibility (estimated by the National Blood Transfusion Service as being less than one chance in a million) that blood may have been donated by an infected person who has yet to develop antibodies – there being a delay between the point at which infection takes place and the production of antibodies (see Section 3.1). To guard against this, people who have been at risk of HIV infection are routinely advised against giving blood. In a very few parts of the world, blood is still not screened in this way, so people who are offered transfusions abroad will have to weigh up the risks involved.

Blood products such as the clotting factors Factor 8 and Factor 9 used by haemophiliacs have also in the past been contaminated by HIV. As a result, a number of haemophiliacs have acquired HIV infection. Depending on the source of the blood products, 60–90% of those using Factor 8 have been affected (Hollan *et al*, 1985) and 0–40% of those using Factor 9 (Goedert *et al*, 1985). These blood products are now routinely treated to render them safe (Rouzioux *et al*, 1985; Felding *et al*, 1985; Meer *et al*, 1986), although one study has disputed the effectiveness of some of the procedures used (White *et al*, 1986).

HIV can also be transmitted if injecting drug users share syringes, needles and other equipment. A detailed discussion of the issues involved here can be found in Chapter 7.

Transmission via organ transplants   HIV has been isolated from body organs, and prior to the HIV antibody testing of donors, transplants were a probable route of transmission. Evidence of transmission via organ transplants has come from cases involving kidney transplants (L'Age-Stehr, *et al*, 1985) and skin grafts (Clark, 1987). All potential donors are now tested for HIV antibodies.

Transmission from mother to child before and around birth   HIV can be transmitted from mother to child before and around birth in a number of ways. Before birth, HIV may be transmitted across the placenta to the developing foetus. During birth, the virus may be transmitted via the mother's blood or perhaps via vaginal and cervical secretions, and after birth there is some, albeit controversial, evidence for transmission via breast milk. It is difficult to distinguish between infection before birth and infection during birth itself since, even if the child is unaffected, it may carry maternal antibodies for some time after being born. These make it difficult to determine the child's own antibody status.

Studies of transmission prior to birth suggest that 30–50% of infants born of seropositive mothers will be infected before birth (Pinching & Jefferies, 1985; Semprini *et al*, 1987; Hicks, 1987). There is also some evidence to suggest that women who have developed an HIV-related illness are more likely than those who are symptomless to pass on infection to their children before birth (Embree *et al*, 1987).

There has been some debate about the value of Caesarean section as a means of delivering children born to HIV-positive mothers. An early study comparing seven children of seropositive mothers who were vaginally delivered with five equivalent children delivered by Caesarean section, revealed that none of the children born by Caesarean section acquired HIV infection whereas three of the vaginally delivered children did (Chiodi, 1986). Subsequent research has suggested that the evidence is less clear cut than this, and while Caesarean section may be associated with a lower risk of HIV infection, infected children may still be born this way (Lapointe, 1985).

HIV, along with other retroviruses, has been isolated from breast milk

(Thiry, 1985), and the first case of HIV infection to take place as the likely consequence of feeding breast milk was reported by Ziegler *et al* (1985). Two other cases have since been reported. In each of these cases, the mother had been infected after the birth of the child, probably via blood transfusions. In 1985, the Centers for Disease Control in Atlanta, USA advised HIV-positive mothers not to breast feed, a recommendation which has since caused considerable controversy.

It is important that the risks associated with breast milk are weighed against the benefits that this may have for mother and child (Baumslag, 1987). Mothers with HIV infection will need to consider carefully with their doctor and other health professionals the advantages and disadvantages of feeding their children in this way.

How HIV is not transmitted

Transmission studies strongly suggest that HIV cannot be transmitted via the following routes:

touch	towels
bodily contact	toilet seats
coughing and sneezing	pets
cups, cutlery and food	mosquitoes and other insects
swimming pools	sharing baths and showers
drinking from the same glass	

There is *no* evidence that HIV can be transmitted through non-sexual contact in households. In a recent study of 90 children of 45 people with AIDS, not one of the children was found to be infected by HIV in spite of the fact that they had regularly hugged and kissed their parents and had shared kitchen and bathroom facilities with them (Fischi *et al*, 1987). In this same study, not one of the 29 friends and relatives living with the people concerned became infected.

There is no evidence either that HIV can be transmitted by close physical contact at the place of work. Indeed, even when health care workers have been accidentally and directly exposed to the virus, the chance of transmission is slight. Of 150 health care workers in the UK who were accidentally exposed to the blood or body fluids of patients infected with HIV, not one sero-converted after a follow-up lasting twelve months (McEvoy & Porter, 1987). In America, where several thousand health care workers have been monitored in this way, only three known cases of sero-conversion have taken place. These involved contact with substantial quantities of blood (*Lancet*, 1987). It cannot be emphasised too strongly that there is no occupational risk in employment where there is no direct contact with the blood, semen and other body fluids of infected individuals. In employment where this does take place, the 'good working practices' that guard against more infectious viruses being transmitted by these same routes (for example, hepatitis B) will be just as effective against HIV.

A considerable amount of popular concern has been expressed about transmission via saliva. Apart from the fact that a quite different profile of infection would be found it this were the case, with family members, household contacts and even casual acquaintances being infected, research has shown that saliva contains at least two components which actually inhibit HIV (Fultz, 1986). Transmission by this route has not been shown to take place.

2.6 THEORETICAL RISKS — THE 'WHAT IF' SYNDROME

Just as a distinction can be made between the contexts from which a virus can be isolated and the contexts in which it can be transmitted, there is a difference between the modes of transmission that are theoretically possible and those that actually take place. In helping others clarify the ways in which HIV is, and is not, transmitted, health educators frequently encounter the 'what if' syndrome, as anxious people conjure up scenarios often based on sensationalist media reporting of events.

In particular, the advent of HIV infection and AIDS has forced a recognition of the diversity of human sexuality and has made it necessary to speak frankly about sexual behaviours that had hitherto been little talked about. It has provided opportunities for people to articulate their personal fears about a wide range of issues to do with sex and sexuality. Health educators therefore need to encourage others to examine their feelings in a non-judgemental way in order to try to identify their underlying causes. Unfortunately, many of those who have deep-rooted anxieties about sexual matters are unlikely to be convinced by rational arguments. They may need time and continuing support to think through the issues involved.

Groundless but real fears concerning the remotest imaginable routes of infection have already led some to nervous breakdowns and even suicide.

Some of the 'worried well' may have a history of repeated HIV antibody testing, and require expert and experienced long-term counselling to help them identify the basis of their fears and anxieties. Cases like these reflect badly on the continued irresponsibility of sections of the mass media for publishing conflicting, sensationalist and misleading reports about HIV transmission.

References

Adler, M. (1987) The development of the epidemic, in M. Adler (ed.) *The ABC of AIDS*, London, *British Medical Journal.*

Amman, A. J. *et al* (1983) Acquired immunodeficiency in an infant: possible transmission by means of blood products, *Lancet*, **i**, pp 956–8.

Barker, D. & Rose, G. (1984) *Epidemiology in Medical Practice*, Edinburgh, Churchill Livingstone.

Baumslag, N. (1987) Breast feeding and HIV infection, *Lancet*, **ii**, p 400.

Bloor, M., Samphier, M. & Prior, L. (1987) Artefact explanations of inadequacies in health: an assessment of the evidence, *Sociology of Health and Illness*, **9**, 3, pp 231–264.

Boffey, P. (1988) Spread of AIDS abating but deaths will still soar, *New York Times*, 14 February, p 36.

Boyton, R. & Scambler, G. (1988) Survey of general practitioners' attitudes to AIDS in the North West Thames and East Anglian regions, *British Medical Journal*, **296**, 20 February.

Calabrese, L. H. & Gopalakrishna, K. U. (1986) Transmission of HTLV-III infection from man to woman to man, *New England Journal of Medicine*, **314**, p 987.

Chiodi, F. *et al* (1986) Vertical transmission of HTLV-III, *Lancet*, **ii**, p 1276.

Clark, J. A. (1987) HIV transmission and skin grafts, *Lancet*, **i**, p 983.

DHSS (1988) Press Release, Quarterly figures on AIDS, 11 January.

Embree, J. *et al* (1987) Does prenatal human immunodeficiency virus infection produce infant malformations? Abstract, 3rd International Conference on AIDS, Washington DC, June.

Esteban, J. *et al* (1985) Importance of Western Blot analysis in predicting infectivity of anti-HTLV-III/LAV positive blood, *Lancet*, **i**, p 1033.

Felding, P. *et al* (1985) Absence of antibodies to LAV/HTLV-III in haemophiliacs with heat-treated factor VIII concentrate of American origin, *Lancet*, **ii**, p 832–3.

Fischi, M. *et al* (1987) Evaluation of heterosexual partners, children and household contacts of adults with AIDS, *Journal of the American Medical Association*, **257**, 5.

Fultz, P. N. (1986) Components of saliva inactivate HIV, *Lancet*, **ii**, p 1215.

Goedert, J. J. *et al* (1985) Antibodies reactive with Human T-cell Leukaemia viruses (HTLV-III) in the sera of haemophiliacs receiving factor 8 concentrate, *Blood*, **65**, p 492–5.

HEA (1989) *AIDS-UK* 6, London, Health Education Authority.

Hicks, C. (1987) Innocent victims, *Nursing Times*, **83** (7), p 19.

Hollan, S. R. *et al* (1985) Immunological alterations in anti HTLV-III negative haemophiliacs and homosexual men in Hungary, *Immunology Letter*, **11**, pp 305–10.

Kingsley, L. *et al* (1987) Risk factors for seroconversion to Human Immunodeficiency Virus amongst male homosexuals, *Lancet*, **i**, pp 345–9.

L'Age-Stehr, J. *et al* (1985) HTLV-III infection in kidney transplant recipients, *Lancet*, **ii**, pp 1361–2.

Lancet (1987) HIV transmission via skin and mucous membranes, *Lancet*, **i**, p 1329.

Lapointe, N. *et al* (1985) Transplacental transmission of HTLV-III virus, *New England Journal of Medicine*, **321**, pp 1325–6.

McCormick, A. (1988) Trends in mortality statistics in England and Wales with particular reference to AIDS from 1984 to April 1987, *British Medical Journal*, **296**, pp 1289–92.

McEvoy, M. & Porter, K. (1987) Health care workers and the risk of HIV infection, *Lancet*, **i**, p 224.

Mann, J. (1988) Introductory address to the World Summit of Ministers of Health on programmes for AIDS prevention, London, 26 January.

Marmor, M. *et al* (1986) Possible female to female transmission of HIV, *Ann Intern Med.*, **105**, p 969.

Meer, J. *et al* (1986) Absence of antibodies to LAV/HTLV-III in haemophiliacs intensively treated with heat-treated factor VIII concentrate, *British Medical Journal*, **292**, p 1049.

Monzon, O. T. & Capellan, J. B. M. (1987) Female-to-female transmission of HIV, *Lancet*, **ii**, p 40-1.

Moss, A. R. (1988) Seropositivity for HIV and the development of AIDS or AIDS related condition: three-year follow-up of the San Francisco General Hospital Cohort, *British Medical Journal*, **295**, pp 745-50.

Pinching, A. J. and Jefferies, D. (1985) AIDS and HTLV-III/LAV infection: consequences for obstetrics and perinatal medicine, *British Journal of Obstetrics and Gynaecology*, **92**, pp 1211-17.

Prior, L. (1985) Making sense of mortality, *Sociology of Health and Illness*, **7, 2**, pp 167-90.

Rouzioux, C. *et al* (1985) Absence of antibodies to AIDS virus in haemophiliacs treated with heat-treated factor VIII concentrate, *Lancet*, **i**, 271-2.

Semprini, A. *et al* (1987) HIV infection and AIDS in newborn babies of mothers positive for HIV antibody, *British Medical Journal*, **294**, p 610.

Stewart, G. J. *et al* (1985) Transmission of Human T-cell Lymphotropic Virus type III (HTLV-III) by artificial insemination by donor, *Lancet*, **ii**, pp 581-4.

Thiry, L. *et al* (1985) Isolation of AIDS virus from cell-free breast milk of three healthy virus carriers, *Lancet*, **ii**, p 891-2.

White, G. C. *et al* (1986) Immunological alterations in anti-HTLV-III seroconversion associated with heat-treated factor VIII concentrate, *Lancet*, **i**, pp 611-12.

WHO (1987) Special Programmme on AIDS, Progress Report No. 2, Geneva, WHO.

Ziegler, J. B. *et al* (1985) Postnatal transmission of AIDS-associated retrovirus from mother to infant, *Lancet*, **i**, pp 896-8.

3.   Tests and testing

It is a common misconception that a simple test can indicate whether someone has AIDS. AIDS is in fact a syndrome of more than thirty distinct life-threatening conditions that can follow HIV infection. Moreover, as we have seen, HIV may have consequences other than AIDS. These include Persistent Generalised Lymphadenopathy (PGL), AIDS-Related Complex (ARC) and symptomless conditions (see Sections 1.1 and 1.2). AIDS therefore is a complex syndrome to identify, and a diagnosis can usually only be made on the basis of the presence of one or more specific opportunistic diseases *in addition* to HIV infection. Logically therefore, there can be no one test which will determine whether or not someone has AIDS. The so-called 'AIDS tests' are in fact not tests for AIDS but for HIV infection or, more correctly, for antibodies to HIV infection.

3.1   THE HIV ANTIBODY TEST

The body often produces antibodies in response to infection by a virus. These antibodies usually neutralise the virus. In the case of HIV infection, however, the antibodies produced are generally unable to neutralise the virus. As a result, the damage caused by the virus goes unchecked, and the affected person can pass on the infection to others.

There are now a number of reliable tests for antibodies to HIV. They can be arranged by a GP or a doctor working in a Sexually Transmitted Diseases (STD) clinic and involve testing a small sample of blood taken usually from a vein in the arm. Results are usually available in two to three weeks. More rarely, an HIV antibody test may be performed in a medical emergency or during in-patient treatment in hospital. In these circumstances, a result can normally be obtained within a few hours. If a test shows the presence of HIV antibodies, the person is said to have seroconverted and to be *antibody positive* (or HIV+). If no antibodies to HIV can be found, a person is said to be *antibody negative* (or HIV-).

What the test reveals

A positive test result reveals that a person has produced antibodies to HIV infection. A negative test result reveals that at the time of testing a person has not developed antibodies to HIV. Although 'false positive' or 'false negative' results sometimes occur, the HIV antibody tests in common use in the UK are now reported to be over 99% accurate in determining whether or not antibodies are present.

What the test does not reveal
A positive result does not reveal whether a person will develop PGL, ARC or AIDS, at least in the short term. Predictions of the proportion of those infected who will subsequently develop one of these conditions vary considerably. For example, estimates of the proportion of people who will develop AIDS in the three-year period following infection currently vary between 8% and 34% (Melbye *et al*, 1987).

A negative test result does not necessarily mean that an individual has *not* been infected, since there can be a delay, varying from a matter of weeks to three months (and occasionally longer) between infection and the production of antibodies. This delay, which has been described as the 'window of uncertainty', raises questions about the appropriateness of a single HIV antibody test as a measure of an individual's HIV status. Those who have been at risk of HIV infection and who obtain a negative result on first testing are therefore often advised to have a repeat test three months later in order to check the original result.

3.2 THE HIV ANTIGEN TEST
The HIV antigen test detects parts of the virus itself rather than antibodies to it. Most of the commercially available antigen tests detect the presence or absence of the core protein p24. It is also possible (although expensive and time-consuming) to test for the whole virus using HIV culture tests (Mortimer 1987).

What the test reveals
The antigen test reveals if someone has been infected by HIV. A growing body of opinion now suggests that the results of an antigen test may also be particularly useful in identifying early infection before antibodies have had a chance to develop (Ranki *et al*, 1987) and in predicting the likely course of infection (Wall *et al* , 1987; Stute, 1987).

What the test does not reveal
The antigen test does not reveal with any certainty whether an infected person will subsequently develop PGL, ARC, AIDS or any other HIV-related illness. There is as yet some unresolved debate about whether an antigen test is a more reliable indicator of HIV infection than an antibody test. While an antigen test may be a more sensitive way of detecting HIV infection in its early stages, when antibody levels may be low, there may be periods following the production of antibodies when viral components cannot be detected.

3.3 ISSUES TO BE CONSIDERED BEFORE TAKING A TEST
Since antibody testing is currently much more common than antigen testing, the following discussion focuses primarily on issues to be considered before deciding whether or not to take an HIV antibody test. Making the decision to

have an HIV antibody test may involve many financial, moral and social considerations. In particular, people will need to consider carefully the implications of receiving either a positive or a negative test result. Ideally, they should do this with the help of a trained counsellor who has experience of HIV testing.

Possible consequences of receiving a negative test result
As has been said, a negative result does not necessarily mean that a person is uninfected. HIV antibodies may not yet have had time to develop. A second test about three months after the first may be advisable if the person concerned has been at risk of HIV infection.

For some people, a negative test result may be a relief as well as the chance to reassess present and future relationships. In the light of a negative result, decisions may be made about the adoption of safer sexual practices (see Chapter 6), about the kinds of relationships that are felt most desirable, and about the appropriateness of past patterns of behaviour.

People receiving a negative result should also be aware that they may be required to declare this in connection with future applications for life insurance. A number of insurance companies have indicated that they may wish to ask people with negative test results a series of supplementary questions about their lifestyles before making the decision whether or not to issue a policy.

It should be recognised, however, that for some of those who are highly anxious about possible HIV infection, even a repeatedly negative test result may offer little or no reassurance. In this kind of situation, sustained counselling and support may be necessary.

Possible consequences of receiving a positive test result
For the majority of people, receiving the news that they are HIV antibody positive is a very distressing experience. No matter how well someone has prepared themselves for this kind of result, its arrival is almost certain to involve some degree of shock. This is the case in spite of the fact that a positive result can sometimes bring relief from the uncertainty of not knowing what the outcome of the test would be. Individual reactions to a positive test result vary widely, from numbness or disbelief to anger, crying and fear.

In the medium to long term, people who have received a positive test result may feel that they have lost control over their lives. They may also experience a loss of self-esteem, occupational disruption, anxiety and depression. In extreme circumstances, these feelings can be so severe as to result in suicidal feelings or suicide itself, but with appropriate support, many of these reactions can lead to more positive outcomes.

In some circumstances, a positive test result accompanied by sensitive counselling may provide much needed reassurance, and encourage the radical reappraisal of priorities and, perhaps, relationships. This too can have positive or negative consequences. Some people may as a result of this take better care of their health generally, something which can be important in enhancing the quality of life after diagnosis. Others may be encouraged to adopt and promote safer sexual practices. On the other hand, a positive test result can occasionally lead to the break up of an existing relationship, perhaps as a result of efforts to apportion blame.

As with a negative result, there is the issue of insurance to consider. In May 1987, the Association of British Insurers recommended that its 425 member companies should question applicants for life insurance about AIDS. Subsequently, all insurance companies in Britain (although not in parts of the United States where state legislation in some cases prevents this from happening) have sought to deny cover to applicants who knowingly have HIV infection. Similar restrictions now apply to health care insurance as well as that taken out for travel overseas.

Finally, there are the likely reactions of others to think about. AIDS and HIV infection are still poorly understood by most people. While there have been widespread programmes of public information in Britain, many people still obtain their knowledge about AIDS from the popular press, whose reporting of the issues has, often, been far from accurate (Wellings, 1988). Parents, spouses, families, lovers, colleagues at work and friends cannot necessarily be relied on to react supportively and appropriately to the news that someone is HIV antibody positive. Health education about AIDS has a crucial role to play in changing attitudes to the syndrome, but until this has happened, care will be needed in breaking the news to others and in anticipating their likely reactions.

3.4 CONFIDENTIALITY

Disclosing the results of an HIV test or even the fact that an HIV test has taken place can have wide-ranging consequences. Confidentiality is therefore crucial. While members of the medical profession are bound to keep information about their patients confidential from the general public, they may feel it appropriate under certain circumstances to share this information with other professional colleagues. While there is a clear practical and moral basis for the confidentiality that exists between a doctor and patient, the legal foundations of this relationship are less sure. Legal rights to confidentiality within the medical profession are based on common law or contracts which, in the final instance, may depend upon a 'court's view of the moral obligation of the physician'. (Talbot, 1986). In certain circumstances, a Crown Court judge may compel a doctor to break patient confidentiality. There may also be cases where the doctor has a statutory duty, as is the case under the Infectious Diseases Act, to disclose information to others. A doctor may also feel at liberty to break confidence if she or he feels in good faith that to do so would be of benefit to the patient.

Many HIV tests currently take place in STD clinics. Ever since the Venereal Diseases Regulations of 1916, confidentiality within these has been to some extent protected by law. These regulations, last updated in 1974, do however allow a doctor to communicate information to another 'medical practitioner or to a person employed under the authority of a medical practitioner in connection with the treatment of persons suffering from such disease for the prevention of the spread thereof and . . . for the purpose of such treatment and prevention' (NHS [Venereal Diseases] Regulations, 1974). Moreover, the DHSS's draft code on the confidentiality of personal health information, produced after the introduction of the Data Protection Act, permits computer-recorded medical information to be disclosed to an 'officer of the health authority' (Talbot, 1986).

The issue of confidentiality continues to be hotly debated within the medical profession itself, with some taking the view that GPs in particular should be routinely informed of the results of HIV tests carried out in STD clinics. Other doctors are opposed to such measures on the grounds that they might create dangerous precedents as well as damage the traditional confidentiality of the doctor-patient relationship.

3.5   HIV TESTING, SCREENING AND CONSENT

There has been much discussion about the value of screening for HIV infection. Screening involves the examination of entire populations or groups within the population for evidence of infection. It can take place anonymously if data is not kept on the identities of those who are tested or it can take place in such a way that infected individuals can be identified. The term 'screening' should not be confused with 'testing' which is the process used to determine the infection or disease status of an individual (WHO/SPA, 1988).

Mass screening

Strong arguments for anonymous screening have been put forward by some doctors who suggest that this is the only way in which to obtain accurate estimates of the prevalence of infection (Peto, 1988; Connor & Kingman, 1988). Others have favoured non-anonymous screening on the grounds that it might enable those with HIV infection to be identified and perhaps segregated. In this particular context, there have been demands for the compulsory (and non-anonymous) testing of either the entire population, or specific groups of individuals. Those who favour this latter course of action argue that people can not be trusted to safeguard their own health and that of others, and society should intervene to prevent the further spread of infection. Demands such as these are frequently linked to the idea that AIDS should be made a notifiable disease. Some have gone so far as to suggest that people with HIV infection should be tattooed or that identification cards should be issued, indicating whether or not a person is free of infection.

These demands frequently show a misunderstanding of what HIV testing can achieve. They assume, for example, that tests are 100% reliable and that the 'window of uncertainty' remains more or less constant. They also make the assumption that all would come forward (or could be found) for testing and that the epidemic would not be driven underground. The financial costs of mass screening without consent would be considerable, as would be the threat to civil liberties. Governments around the world have resisted calls for compulsory testing and in late 1987, the Council of Europe issued a statement making it clear that the compulsory testing of the general population or of particular groups could not under any circumstances be condoned.

Pregnancy

There have also been demands for screening which claim to have their origins in a concern for the needs of people with HIV infection themselves. It has been suggested that the early detection of disease may lead to more effective medical intervention and treatment. Recent debate has centred on the desirability (or otherwise) of the routine testing of women who are pregnant. Concern of this kind was first voiced following reports that pregnancy might lead to the development of AIDS in women with HIV infection (Pinching & Jefferies, 1985; Minkoff, 1986). Subsequent research has questioned the validity of these findings (Ciraru-Vigneron *et al*, 1987) on the grounds that atypical groups of women with HIV infection may have been studied, and it is at present unclear what role pregnancy plays in the development of AIDS in women with HIV infection. In this situation, it is vital that women are offered appropriate counselling and that their right to decide whether or not to have a test is protected.

Another consideration for women who are HIV antibody positive and who are pregnant is the risk of transmitting HIV to the foetus. A number of studies suggest that the likelihood of this happening may be anything up to 50 and 60%. While it is too early to say for sure how many children born with HIV will subsequently develop AIDS, a mortality rate of 61% has been recorded by some researchers (Loveman *et al*, 1986).

Given this kind of evidence, there have been calls for the compulsory testing of pregnant women, and in Scotland there have already been trials involving the routine testing of women perceived to be from 'high-risk groups'. In July 1987, however, the Royal College of Midwives rejected demands for mandatory testing, suggesting that women who may have been at risk should be encouraged instead to give their informed consent to the procedure.

Doctors and patients

Issues of consent have arisen not only within the context of demands for the screening of the entire population or specified groups but also within discussion about the rights of doctors and patients. In 1987, following a heated debate about such issues in a number of medical journals, the British Medical Association's (BMA) annual conference debated whether doctors should have the right to administer HIV tests without consent. A resolution was passed which stated that testing should take place at the discretion of the patient's doctor and should not necessarily require the consent of the patient. This resolution has subsequently generated extensive debate both within the BMA and elsewhere. The Medical Defence Union has subsequently criticised the resolution on the grounds that doctors pursuing this course of action might render themselves liable to legal prosecution on the charge of abuse to the person. The United Kingdom Central Council (UKCC) has made it clear to nurses that to 'knowingly collude' with a doctor in obtaining blood specimens for HIV testing without consent could lay them open to the charge of aiding and abetting assault. Subsequently, the BMA's council has decided not to implement the resolution. It is, however, important for those who do not wish an HIV test to be carried out to make this clear to a medical practitioner carrying out a series of tests for which consent in general terms has been given.

In late 1987, demands were voiced concerning the rights of patients to know whether or not their doctor was infected, and in December of that year, the General Medical Council issued a statement which made it clear that doctors who consider that they might be HIV positive should seek diagnostic testing and counselling. Those found to be HIV positive should seek specialist advice regarding the most appropriate steps to take to ensure that infection is not passed on to others through their professional practice.

3.6   HIV TESTING AND EMPLOYMENT

In a series of statements, the DHSS has clearly repeated that there is no risk of HIV infection at work where there is no direct contact with the blood, semen or other body fluids of infected individuals. This view is entirely in line with what is known about the ways in which HIV can be transmitted (see Section 2.5). Few jobs involve coming into contact with these fluids, and the vast majority of employees are therefore safe from infection whilst at work (Department of Employment/Health and Safety Executive, 1987). A number of trade unions and professional associations have now issued guidelines for their members spelling out what constitutes 'good working practice'. These include the BMA, the RCN, COHSE, NUPE, NALGO and various teaching unions.

The advent of HIV infection has provided an important opportunity for employers to review the extent to which established 'good practice' is adhered to on their premises. A number of commentators have suggested that prior to the epidemic, standards in some organisations may have been less than satisfactory in this respect.

Established 'good practice' within the context of first aid is quite sufficient. When giving mouth-to-mouth resuscitation, it may be useful to employ a special mouthpiece, but it should be noted that no cases of infection have been reported as a result of giving mouth-to-mouth resuscitation without such equipment. The 'kiss of life' therefore should never be withheld simply because a mouthpiece is not available.

There is no reason why someone with HIV infection should not continue to work so long as they are medically fit to do so; only rarely would a move to alternative duties be appropriate. Similarly, there is no reason to treat people with HIV infection differently from others when considering them as applicants for employment. The DHSS has stated that it is inappropriate to require employees to disclose their HIV status or to submit to tests for the virus — a position echoed by a recent statement from the Council of Europe (Council of Europe, 1987). Employers considering introducing HIV testing for employees do so contrary to all the available scientific and medical evidence.

Given inaccurate and sensationalist media portrayals of AIDS, it is not surprising that some employees may be unduly anxious about working with those who have HIV infection. Health education in the workplace may be needed in order to counteract unreasonable fears and anxieties. Ideally, this should take place before someone is thought to be infected.

Sadly, there have already been cases of individuals being dismissed from work on the grounds that they are HIV positive. Some of these have taken place after employees have refused to work alongside those who are infected. Actions of this kind are not only grossly unjust, they may also fuel the groundless fears of others by suggesting that there is an occupational risk associated with HIV infection.

3.7 TESTING, IMMIGRATION AND BORDER CONTROL

A number of countries have introduced immigration restrictions designed to deny permanent residence to those with HIV infection or AIDS. A few countries have also considered imposing restrictions on tourism and short-stay visits. Up-to-date information about these can be obtained from the embassies and consulates of the countries concerned and also from the National AIDS Helpline (see Appendix C).

It should be recognised, however, that discrepancies can often arise between the stated policy of a government and the practices of its border and immigration officials.

In considering the appropriateness of border control as a means of restricting the international movement of those with HIV infection, the Council of Europe has recently issued a statement that control measures at borders are scientifically and ethically unjustifiable (Council of Europe, 1987). WHO has also published an extensive report on the question of international travel and HIV infection. It points out that since no region in the world is free from HIV infection and AIDS, and given our understanding of HIV's modes of transmission, 'it makes little sense in public health terms, to undertake screening of international travellers using clinical aspects of AIDS as criteria for exclusion.'

Moreover, because of the 'window of uncertainty' between infection and the production of antibodies, HIV antibody tests will not identify a newly infected person even though she or he may be capable of transmitting the virus. WHO concludes that 'HIV screening programmes for international travellers would, at best and at *great cost*, retard *only briefly* the dissemination of HIV both globally and with respect to any particular country' (WHO, 1987). This conclusion is entirely in keeping with the 'Declaration on AIDS Prevention' made at the World Summit of Ministers of Health in London in January 1988.

These statements have important implications in relation to proposals for the screening of international travellers. Deficiencies in the test sensitivities will mean that some HIV-positive individuals will not be detected in addition to those who go undetected because of the 'window' effect. This will seriously affect the predictive value of test results.

In this situation where demands are made that travellers be screened for HIV antibodies, it may be particularly important to consider the degree of confidence we can have in a positive test result. WHO (1987) has pointed out:

'Consider a cohort of 1,000,000 travellers, among whom 1% (10,000) are truly HIV positive and 99% (990,000) are negative. If the serological screening test has a sensitivity (accuracy in identifying true positives) of 99%, then 9,900 of the 10,000 true positives would be identified and 100 would be undetected (false negatives). If the serological test has a specificity (accuracy in identifying true negatives) of 99%, then of the total 990,000 true negatives, this test would correctly identify 980,100 but would label 9,900 negatives as falsely positive. Thus of the total 19,800 'positives' identified by the screening of this population, half are true positives and half are false positives. The positive predictive value of the screening test in this situation would be 50%. In addition, 100 true positive (HIV infected) persons would be falsely identified as negative. Therefore, even a test of very high sensitivity and specificity can lead to a massive misallocation of resources in response to false-positive individuals, while allowing some truly positive individuals to remain undetected. In practice, sensitivity and specificity may fall below 99%, especially in busy laboratories lacking adequate resources of equipment, skilled staff, supervision and quality control'.

References

Ciraru-Vigneron, N. *et al* (1987) HIV infection among high risk pregnant women, *Lancet*, **i**, p 630.

Connor, S. & Kingman, S. (1988) The trouble with testing, *New Scientist*, 28 January, pp 60–3.

Council of Europe (1987) Recommendation No. R(87), 25 November.

Department of Employment/Health and Safety Executive (1987) *AIDS and Employment*, London, Department of Employment.

Loveman, A. *et al* (1986) AIDS in pregnancy, *Journal of Gynaecology and Neonatal Nursing*, **15**, pp 91–3.

Melbye, M. *et al* (1987) The natural history of human immunodeficiency virus infection, in M.S. Gottlieb *et al* (eds) *Current Topics in AIDS*, Vol. 1, ch. 4, Chichester, John Wiley.

Minkoff, H.L. (1986) AIDS. Time for obstetricians to get involved, *Obstetrics and Gynaecology*, **68**, pp 267–8.

Mortimer, P. (1987) The virus and the tests, in M. Adler (ed) *ABC of AIDS*, London, British Medical Journal.

NHS (Venereal Diseases) Regulations (1974) London, HMSO.

Peto, J. (1988) The case for HIV testing, *New Scientist*, 26 January, p 23.

Pinching, A. & Jefferies, D. (1985) AIDS and HTLV-III/LAV infection: consequences for obstetrics and perinatal medicine, *British Journal of Obstetrics and Gynaecology*, **92**, pp 1211–17.

Ranki, A. *et al* (1987) Long latency precedes over sero-conversion in sexually transmitted HIV infection, *Lancet*, **ii**, pp 589–93.

Stute, R. (1987) HIV antigen detection in routine blood donor screening, *Lancet*, **i**, p 566.

Talbot, M.D. (1986) Confidentially – the law in England, *Genito-urinary Medicine*, **62**, **4**, pp 270–6.

Wall, R.A. *et al* (1987) HIV antigen anaemia in acute HIV infection, *Lancet*, **i**, p 566.

Wellings, K. (1988) Perceptions of risk – media treatment of AIDS, in P. Aggleton and H. Homans (eds) *Social Aspects of AIDS*, Lewes, Falmer Press.

WHO (1987) Report of the consultation on international travel and HIV infection, Geneva, WHO.

WHO/SPA (1988) *Screening and Testing in AIDS Prevention and Control Programmes*, Geneva, WHO.

4.   Lay beliefs about HIV infection and AIDS

There are many ways of explaining health, illness and disease. Some of these are scientific and emphasise the role that viruses and bacteria can play in causing disease. Others are closer to the folklore and common sense that people use to make sense of their everyday lives. It is often said that you can catch a cold by sitting in a draught, by not wrapping up well when going out or by not drying your hair properly after washing it. These popular explanations are sometimes called *lay beliefs* about health. They have their origins in shared cultural experiences such as superstition, religion and politics which invariably interact with more scientific understandings of health issues. The media too plays an important role in generating and sustaining powerful images of illness, disability and sexuality.

Lay beliefs about health are not always inaccurate; they sometimes contain elements of truth. Thus the lay belief that strain and worry is the main cause of 'stomach' disease may be at least partly true because there is a relationship between stress and the onset of gastric and duodenal ulcers. Doctors and other health professionals subscribe to lay beliefs about health and disease. For example, Helman's (1978) research in general practice suggests that many doctors share the lay belief that cough mixtures and hot drinks may be helpful in 'flushing out' and 'shifting' the germs that cause chest infections.

4.1   WHY ARE LAY BELIEFS IMPORTANT?

Lay beliefs can also encourage people to misperceive the risks associated with particular kinds of behaviour. Evidence from research into tobacco and alcohol use suggests that lay beliefs about health are very important in determining whether or not a person responds to conventional health education. For example, even though people may know that excessive smoking endangers their health, they may continue to smoke forty cigarettes a day 'safe' in the belief that only a susceptible few subsequently develop lung cancer. Within the context of HIV infection, the belief that AIDS only affects gay men and injecting drug users may similarly result in some people misperceiving the risks associated with particular sexual acts.

Lay beliefs about health may weaken the effects of health education campaigns which emphasise medical information. Compared with lay health knowledge, scientific 'facts' and 'theories' may seem distant and removed to many people. Doctors are now increasingly aware of the need to bring their explanations of health, illness and disease closer to those of their patients and clients.

Some lay beliefs suggest that illness is a retribution for wrong doing. This frequently results in various kinds of victim blaming. We can see this in the case of the Black Death during the fourteenth century when Jews and Gypsies were blamed for spreading infection. Similar events took place in the nineteenth century when the Irish were blamed for spreading cholera. Health educators will find it useful to anticipate the lay beliefs that different groups share when planning their health education initiatives.

4.2   RESEARCH INTO LAY BELIEFS ABOUT HIV INFECTION AND AIDS

There has been considerable medical and scientific research into HIV infection and AIDS, as well as into the extent to which different groups are acquainted with the medical facts. However, few studies have systematically examined people's lay beliefs about HIV infection and AIDS. Research is now underway into the lay health beliefs of gay men (Boulton, Fitzpatrick & Hart, 1988), undergraduate students (Clift & Stears, 1988) and young people participating in local authority youth provision and youth training schemes (Warwick, Aggleton & Homans, 1988). Findings from some of these studies can be found in *AIDS: Social Representations and Social Practices* (Aggleton, Hart & Davies, 1989).

4.3   LAY BELIEFS ABOUT HIV INFECTION AND AIDS

There are several different kinds of lay belief about HIV infection and AIDS. First, there are beliefs about AIDS itself, what it is and how it can be diagnosed. Second, there are lay beliefs which 'explain' the origins of AIDS. Third, there are lay beliefs which 'explain' why some people develop AIDS and others do not. Fourth, there are lay beliefs which identify the people, the situations and the activities that are perceived as particularly risky. Finally, there are lay beliefs which distinguish between supposedly 'innocent' and 'guilty' victims of infection. These five kinds of lay belief are significant because they help people build up a particular image of AIDS. They are also important because they may influence how individuals respond to health education.

Beliefs about AIDS

It has long been known that the language used to talk about a particular phenomenon dramatically affects the way in which it is thought about as well as the responses that are made to it. Later, issues to do with language and sexuality (see Section 6.2) and language and injecting drug use are examined for these reasons. Our understanding of injecting drug use, for example, is likely to be influenced a great deal by whether someone is said to be an 'injecting drug user', an injecting drug abuser an 'addict' or a 'junkie' (see Section 7.1). Considerations like these also apply when we talk about health issues, since the language used to describe these says much about the way in which that issue is widely understood. Nowhere is this more evident than in everyday talk about HIV infection and AIDS. If we listen carefully to the way doctors and lay people talk about the syndrome as well as about those who are infected and those who are not, it is possible to learn much about the interface between 'folk knowledge' about HIV infection and AIDS and the medical facts (Silverman, 1989).

Perhaps the most important set of lay beliefs about the nature of AIDS comes from the notion that there is an 'AIDS virus'. This immediately leads to confusion between HIV, a virus with well understood modes of transmission, and AIDS, a syndrome of some thirty distinct medical conditions. Moreover, as we have seen, HIV may have many consequences prior to and sometimes independent of AIDS, including PGL and ARC (see Sections 1.1 and 1.2). Talk of an 'AIDS virus' collapses together these crucial distinctions, and presents AIDS as the *cause* of infection, rather than as one of its *outcomes*.

'AIDS carrier' is a similarly misleading term which conjures up a whole series of images about contagion and plague which predate the AIDS pandemic. Its use undermines health education by invoking medically unjustified deep-seated fears about possible contagion. The notion of the 'AIDS carrier' also implies that people with AIDS are *threatening* rather than *threatened*. Furthermore, it makes it difficult for people to distinguish between what it means to have HIV infection, and what it means to have AIDS. Because terms such as 'AIDS virus' and 'AIDS carriers' carry the implication that AIDS can be 'caught' by casual contact, it is important for health educators to avoid using them.

Given the widespread use of these terms within the media and elsewhere, it is perhaps not surprising that 20% of people recently surveyed believed that they could 'catch' AIDS via shared washing, cooking and eating utensils (Campbell & Waters, 1987). Health educators should also recognise that the terms in which the effectiveness of AIDS education is often evaluated may reinforce popular misconceptions. Thus, for example, a New York newspaper has reported that 40% of those whom it had asked thought that AIDS could be 'caught' by giving blood (Moreno, 1987). This poll was based on a single question: 'To the best of your knowledge, can a person catch AIDS by giving blood or not?' Readers were informed that the correct answer was 'No'. However, the only correct answer to this question would require a challenge to the implication that AIDS can be 'caught' at all.

Unfortunately, some kinds of health education have fallen into this same trap, stating that you can't 'catch' AIDS, for example, by sharing a glass of water, by shaking hands and so on. Materials like these fail to question the assumption that AIDS can be 'caught', and subtly reinforce the tendency to discuss HIV and AIDS as if they are identical, and transmitted via casual contact.

The term 'full-blown' AIDS also tends to reinforce the view that AIDS is a unitary phenomenon, rather than a syndrome of a wide variety of medical conditions which may be combined in many different ways. The popular notion of 'full-blown' AIDS also implies that AIDS is the only and inevitable result of HIV infection. It thus obscures the predicament of the large numbers of people with PGL or ARC who may be seriously ill, but are not diagnosed with AIDS itself.

Once views like these become widely established as common sense, it is easy to misunderstand the nature and significance of HIV tests, especially when these are frequently mis-described as 'AIDS tests' (see Chapter 3). No single blood test can detect both HIV and the great variety of opportunistic infections and malignancies that define the Acquired Immune Deficiency Syndrome. Health educators therefore face a considerable task of re-educating those who are likely to think of most aspects of AIDS in the terms outlined above. In this respect, it is particularly important to challenge lay perceptions which regard HIV disease as a death sentence as well as the unhelpful morbidity and fatalism that surrounds the entire subject of AIDS (Watney, 1988).

This inability to distinguish between HIV and AIDS is reflected in the ways in which those affected by HIV or AIDS are often discussed. Thus, we hear frequent talk of 'AIDS victims' and 'AIDS sufferers', terms which reveal much about everyday fears concerning AIDS, but very little about the reality of the syndrome. The category of 'victim' invariably functions to disempower people with a wide variety of illnesses, from cancer to multiple sclerosis, by suggesting that those with incurable illnesses are powerless in the face of disease. This is especially inaccurate when it comes to HIV infection and its various consequences, since many different therapies have been developed to help people with HIV or AIDS improve the quality of their lives (see Section 1.5). It was for exactly these reasons that in 1983 a large number of people with HIV infection, ARC and AIDS met in Denver, Colorado at a National AIDS Forum to produce the *Founding Statement of People With AIDS/ARC*. The Denver Principles state that: 'We condemn attempts to label us as "victims", which implies defeat, and we are only occasionally "patients", which implies passivity, helplessness and dependence on the care of others. We are "people with AIDS" ' (Callen, 1987).

By emphasising the distinction between HIV and AIDS, health educators can increase public awareness of the ways in which the virus is transmitted and help people to assess the degrees of risk arising in their own behaviours. Both these tasks are vital to the successful prevention of HIV infection. Unless people understand precisely what it is that they are at risk from, they cannot be expected to make rational decisions to protect themselves and their sexual partners from possible infection.

To some, this discussion of terminology may seem a matter of semantics. But these are crucial issues to those who live with HIV infection and AIDS. Loose talk which relies heavily on lay perceptions of AIDS has trivialised and sensationalised what are important human, scientific and medical distinctions.

Health educators owe it to those they work with to be clear in their use of terminology and to allay anxiety and fear wherever this is possible, rather than contribute to it.

Beliefs about origins

> When AIDS claimed its first homosexual victims, ordinary people nodded their heads and saw it as God's vengence on those who led unnatural and promiscuous lives.
>
> *The Sun*

Perhaps the most powerful set of lay beliefs about origins are those which suggest AIDS is the consequence of divine retribution. According to this view, AIDS has been unleashed on the world, and upon gay men, prostitutes and injecting drug users in particular, because their actions have infringed a divinely inspired 'natural' social order.

> 'Is AIDS a punishment from God you ask? I would rather call it a warning. Perhaps this frightful illness should make us aware of what's happening in the world. It should show us what happens when moral boundaries fall. I feel that people must reflect more and correct their morals.
>
> Interviewee quoted in the *News of the World*

The idea that disease might be the result of divine intervention or supernatural forces is an old one. In the fourteenth century, for example, the Black Death was popularly understood as a punishment sent from God (Altman, 1986). In the United States, beliefs such as these have been recruited to the service of broader campaigns concerned with 'moral re-armament'. Jerry Falwell, the erstwhile leader of the Moral Majority, has been quoted as saying 'AIDS is the wrath of God against homosexuals' (cited in Altman, 1986) and similar sentiments have been voiced here in Britain. Even were we to accept them on their own terms, beliefs such as these are extraordinary incoherent. As Rabbi Julia Neuberger has said, 'It is a strange God who chooses to punish male homosexuals and not female, and who is angry with drug-takers who inject . . . but not with those who sniff' (Neuberger, 1985). Nevertheless, ideas like these, which run counter to rational and empirical claims, are likely to be particularly powerful filters of health education messages.

Other lay beliefs about origins suggest that AIDS (rarely do lay explanations differentiate between HIV infection and AIDS) might have been manufactured in the research laboratory, perhaps in connection with experiments in genetic engineering or biological warfare. Depending on the person's broader political beliefs, either the CIA or the KGB may be to blame.

A related explanation suggests that AIDS is the consequence of pollution, or the result of ecological instability triggered off by attempts to meddle with the environment.

There are also xenophobic lay beliefs about origins which suggest that AIDS originated in other countries or other communities. Although the first cases of AIDS were diagnosed in the United States and in Europe, these explanations frequently identify an African origin for the syndrome. The isolation of a virus genetically similar in some ways to HIV from African green monkeys has been taken by some as support for this view (Biggar, 1986) as did early reports that HIV antibodies could be isolated from stored Ugandan sera dating back to the early 1970s (Saxinger *et al*, 1985). A discussion of some of the problems associated with the interpretation of these findings can be found in Chirimuuta & Chirimuuta (1987). Rather curiously, the discovery that viruses such as visna (which causes scrapie in sheep) and bovine leukaemia virus share genetic similarities with HIV has done little to affect the popularity of these beliefs. Both of these viruses can be isolated from animals in the United States.

In the light of this, many people find claims about African origins deeply worrying and potentially racist since they feed so easily into stereotypes and prejudices about 'disease', 'black sexuality' and a geographically and socially undifferentiated 'Africa' (Chirimuuta & Chirimuuta, 1987). Lay beliefs about AIDS having an African origin have so informed the common sense of writers of popular and scientific texts about AIDS that, in some books, they are currently presented not as theories about origins but as the truth. Here, as elsewhere, it is important for health educators to challenge arguments which interpret the point of emergence of a virus as its cause. Wherever HIV originated, it is not helpful to hold that region or the people living in it to blame.

Beliefs about causes

Research into lay beliefs about the factors that cause someone to develop AIDS suggests that an important distinction can be made between two sets of ideas. The first of these suggests that AIDS is the result of something within people, the second that AIDS is caused by something outside or around them.

Endogenous beliefs about the cause of AIDS, as we can call the first of these sets of ideas, suggest that AIDS is caused not by a virus but by some quality of the individual or person themselves. According to this point of view, some people may be predisposed to develop AIDS by virtue of their sexuality or their lifestyle. For example, in Vass's (1986) study of public opinion and AIDS carried out in the early stages of the epidemic, it was found that 44% of those interviewed felt that homosexuality in itself was the cause of AIDS. Only 14% were able at that time to identify a viral cause for the syndrome. Such views may be particularly distressing for the families of people with AIDS. More recent research carried out by the British Market Research Bureau for the DHSS suggests that gay men, 'promiscuous' people and injecting drug users are widely perceived to be at special risk of AIDS, regardless of whether they involve themselves in acts that are likely to result in the transmission of the virus (DHSS, 1987).

Closely related to the idea that some individuals may be predisposed to develop AIDS because of the kind of person they are, is the notion that others may somehow be protected from it. There is growing evidence from research carried out in the United States and in Britain that some people believe that by generally keeping fit, by being 'speedy', by being 'aggressively heterosexual', by being 'streetwise' or by leading a 'good Christian life', it is possible to avoid infection.

Another set of lay beliefs of this kind suggests that AIDS can be found endogenously within us all. In work associated with the *Young People's Health Knowledge and AIDS Project,* a number of people were interviewed who believed that AIDS (like cancer so it is suggested) may lurk within all of us. All that is needed in order to 'trigger it off' is the right combination of circumstances (Warwick, Aggleton & Homans, 1988). These events may be either environmental or behavioural in nature. Being overstressed or having 'too much sex' were frequently identified by some of those interviewed as critical ways in which this could come about.

Of a rather different order are exogenous lay beliefs which suggest that the cause of AIDS can be found outside or around the person. Some people believe that AIDS is 'all around us' and that everyone, regardless of their own behaviour, is currently at risk of infection. Ideas like these link closely to the view that being near an infected person is sufficient for transmission to take place — a notion that would seem to have informed the actions of those reported on in the following newspaper items.

Two policemen wore white 'space suits' to guard an AIDS victim in court it was revealed yesterday.

The Sun

'I think that seeing a doctor who has AIDS would be very risky from a health point of view...I would be bloody terrified if I knew my doctor had it, and I'd never go and see him again.'

Interviewee reported in the *News of the World*
following concern about doctors with AIDS, November 1987.

Beliefs about risk

Preliminary findings from research carried out in connection with the *Young People's Health Knowledge and AIDS* project suggest that in assessing the risks to themselves and others, some interviewees emphasise the role that chance and 'bad luck' may play in determining whether or not they become infected

(Warwick, Aggleton & Homans, 1988). Lay beliefs like these are likely to influence the extent to which people feel able to take effective steps to safeguard themselves and others from infection.

Other reports suggest that some people may feel they may be able to minimise the risks by being selective in their choice of prospective sexual partners. In a recent article in *Sunday Magazine,* for example, a young woman discussing whether she would have unprotected sex with someone she met on holiday said she would try to 'wait two weeks and check out a guy really thoroughly' before having sex with him. In the event, her investigations into her prospective partner's social credentials came to an abrupt close after two days when she met a 'nice boy — respectable, well-mannered and well-spoken' (*Sunday Magazine,* 1987). The couple then had penetrative sex without using a condom.

Popular perceptions of risk have been influenced both by media portrayals of AIDS as a disease of social difference (one that affects primarily those who are gay, bisexual, injectors of drugs) and as a disease which has serious and debilitating consequences. These images, which frequently bear little relationship to the realities of HIV infection, may dramatically affect people's judgements about the safety or otherwise of initiating new sexual relationships, especially when the prospective sexual partner shows no sign of disease. In the light of this, health educators will need to devise strategies to help others identify more accurately the risks associated with particular sexual choices (see Chapter 6).

'Innocent' and 'guilty' victims

AIDS: Why must the innocent suffer?

Daily Express

Of course people should not be persecuted or blamed for catching AIDS, because that is vindictive and uncharitable and anyway, it can be caught innocently.

Sunday Telegraph

A final set of lay beliefs about HIV infection and AIDS differentiates between supposedly innocent and guilty victims of infection. Haemophiliacs, blood transfusion recipients, children and the married partners of those who engage in extra-marital relationships are usually termed 'innocent', and gay men, injecting drug users, prostitutes, the 'promiscuous' and bisexuals are usually 'guilty'. These kinds of beliefs often arise not from rational thought but from moral judgements about different kinds of behaviour.

They are also dangerous and divisive since they imply that some people may have 'chosen' to acquire HIV infection. Prostitutes, gay men and injecting drug users come popularly to be seen as having acquired HIV infection as a result of their own fully informed choices. These beliefs fail to recognise that a variety of factors in Britain and elsewhere conspired to ensure that, for some time after the risks associated with injecting drug use, untreated blood products and unprotected sex with an infected person were known about, little systematic health education took place. They also fail to address the complex economic and social factors that sustain female and male prostitution, make injecting drug use a meaningful response for some people and limit the social contexts in which same-sex relationships can be established.

4.4 CONCLUSIONS

Lay beliefs about HIV infection and AIDS have been discussed at length for several reasons. For one thing, there are serious problems with health education programmes which assume that people will find medical and scientific knowledge easy to understand. People are not passive receivers of health education messages. Rather, they actively interpret the information they encounter, shaping it to make it fit in with what they already know. Educators who underestimate the significance of this may think they are providing people with the 'facts' about AIDS when all they may be doing is fuelling popular anxieties, fears, prejudices and stereotypes.

In conclusion, it is important to recognise that lay beliefs about HIV infection and AIDS are not spontaneously generated, but arise from the ways in which people make sense of the information they have access to. Much of this currently comes from media portrayals of AIDS and HIV infection — some of which are misleading and inaccurate. Health educators therefore have a key role to play in helping others evaluate the ways in which the syndrome continues to be popularly portrayed.

References

Aggleton, P.J., Hart, G. & Davies, P.(eds) (1989) *AIDS: Social Representations and Social Practices,* Lewes, Falmer Press.
Altman, D. (1986) *AIDS and the New Puritanism,* London, Pluto Press.
Biggar, R. (1986) The AIDS problem in Africa, *Lancet,* **i,** pp 79–82.
Boulton, M., Fitzpatrick, R. & Hart, G. (1988) Health beliefs and the behaviour of homosexual men. Ongoing project based in the Department of Community Medicine and General Practice, University of Oxford.
Callen, M. (1987) *Surviving and Thriving with AIDS,* New York, GMHC.
Campbell, M. & Waters, W. (1987) Public knowledge about AIDS is increasing, *British Medical Journal,* **294,** pp 892–3.
Chirimuuta, R. & Chirimuuta, R. (1987) *AIDS, Africa and Racism.* Available from R. Chirimuuta, Bretby House, Stanhope, Bretby, Burton on Trent, DE15 0PT.
Clift, S. & Stears, D. (1988) Beliefs and attitudes regarding AIDS among British college students, *Health Education Research,* **3, 1,** pp 75–88.
DHSS (1987) *AIDS: Monitoring response to the public education campaign, February 1986–February 1987,* London, HMSO.
Helman, C. (1978) 'Feed a cold, starve a fever': Folk models of infection in an English suburban community and their relation to medical treatment, *Culture, Medicine and Society,* **2,** pp 107-37
Neuberger, J. (1985) AIDS and the cruelty of panic, *Guardian,* 9 November.
Moreno, S. (1987) Forty per cent think AIDS can be caught by giving blood, *Newsday,* 16 June.
Saxinger, C. *et al* (1985) Unique pattern of HTLV-III (AIDS-related) antigen recognition by sera from African children in Uganda (1972), *Cancer Research,* **45,** (99 Suppl), pp 4624–6.
Silverman, D. (1989) Making sense of a precipice: constituting identity in an HIV clinic, in P.J. Aggleton, G. Hart & P. Davies (eds) *AIDS: Social Representations and Social Practices,* Lewes, Falmer Press.
Sunday Magazine (1987) The young British on holiday, 5 July.
Warwick, I., Aggleton, P.J. & Homans, H. (1988) Young people's beliefs about AIDS, in P.J. Aggleton & H. Homans (eds) *Social Aspects of AIDS,* Lewes, Falmer Press.
Watney, S. (1988) The spectacle of AIDS, *October,* **43.**
Vass, A. (1986) *AIDS: A Plague in Us,* Cambridge, Venus Academica.

5. Sexual lifestyles

This chapter on sexual behaviour and sexual lifestyles aims to prepare health educators for issues that can arise in connection with health education about sexuality, sexual awareness and safer sex. Work in this field requires sensitivity, tact, open-mindedness and a non-judgemental attitude. Moreover, if health educators are to help clients separate fact from fiction, and prejudice from understanding, they will need access to information about sex and sexuality beyond that gained from their own immediate experience. Some may have already participated in courses on sexuality awareness, but for those who are less familiar with the issues this chapter will be of vital importance. Ideally, however, it will need to be complemented by active involvement in workshops and training programmes focusing on sexuality and sexual awareness. Organisations which run courses of this kind, as well as other relevant resources, are listed in Appendix A.

5.1 BACKGROUND

One of the most tenacious misconceptions concerning HIV infection, ARC and AIDS is the belief that the first groups in Britain to be affected by the epidemic were somehow its cause. Just as in the past infectious diseases were commonly attributed to the air, climate or the seasons, so today it is not unusual to regard particular lifestyles as the cause of illness (Herzlich & Pierret, 1986).

This situation is complicated by the fact that the groups with which HIV infection and AIDS have most been associated in Europe and North America are those already held in low regard. The extent to which AIDS continues to be portrayed as the outward sign of an inner moral and sexual turpitude is related to the survival of pre-modern perceptions of health and human sexuality. HIV, like any other virus is no respecter of persons, and in the context of health education, there would be no need to discuss the issue of sexuality at all, beyond the issue of how HIV is transmitted, were it not for the cultural associations that link AIDS with prostitutes, injecting drug users, bisexuals, the 'promiscuous' and in particular gay men.

The discussion of lay beliefs in Chapter 4 has highlighted the tendency to identify particular sexual groups as the *cause* of AIDS, rather than as the first to be affected, and this raises important questions for health education, since it can feed so easily into demands for retribution against particular sections of society.

In reality, HIV can infect anyone, and it has had devastating effects on widely divergent social groups in different parts of the world. An awareness of the different social contexts in which sexual relationships take place is essential for effective health education since, unless we understand what people actually want, like and *do* sexually, we cannot identify successful strategies to minimise the risk of further infection.

5.2   WHAT IS SEX? WHAT IS SEXUALITY?

At first sight it might be considered a little odd to ask questions such as these. After all, doesn't everyone know what sex is? And surely sexuality is something which people either have or they haven't? In fact, there are tremendous variations in the way in which 'sex' is defined. For some people, sex is an act which must involve bodily penetration and orgasm otherwise it is not the 'real thing'. For others, sex is a term which can be used to describe a wider range of experiences which can include touching, holding, caressing or simply being in the presence of someone else. These events may or may not be accompanied by orgasm.

Sexuality is an even more ambiguous term since it can be used to describe the signals that another person gives off — be these looks, smells or ways of behaving — as well as the erotic preferences that someone has.

Most people tend to believe that sex and sexuality are somehow 'natural' and 'inevitable', the result of instinct and animal urges. This is a powerful way of thinking about sex and ourselves in relation to it. But even a quick look at history or at cultural variations around the world will lead us to question such a view. Sexual preferences and patterns of sexual behaviour vary a great deal over time or between cultures.

Nevertheless, it would appear that in any one culture at any one moment, certain forms of sexual expression are valued more highly than others. At the present moment in history (and in British society) there can be little doubt that penetrative vaginal intercourse between one woman and one man is given special priority, in the media and in public discussions about sex, if not within the home. Indeed, sex manuals such as Comfort's (1977) *The Joy of Sex* describe this kind of activity as the 'Main Course', and other forms of sexual expression are relegated to the realm of 'Starters', 'Sauces and Pickles' and 'Problems'. But simply because some forms of sexual expression are given higher priority than others at one particular moment does not mean that other ways of expressing sexuality are less important. When viewed historically and cross-culturally, this tendency to equate 'sex' with penetrative intercourse, whether vaginal or anal, is limiting.

Powerful social forces in politics, religion and even in medicine encourage us to see some sexual acts as more normal than others. But no particular act is intrinsically more 'natural' than any other, it has only been created as such by complex social and cultural processes which may change over time. As Plummer (1986) has noted in this context:

' . . . Human sexuality is thought about, fantasised about, talked about, written about and scripted into action. It is enmeshed in the dialogues of theology, philosophy, medicine, literature, law, morality, psychiatry and the sciences. However biological and "animal like" its foundations may be, human sexuality comes to life through these languages . . . '

Similar ideas to these can also be found in the work of writers such as Ettorre (1980) whose work has focused particularly on what it is to be a lesbian. She has written,

' . . . Lesbianism exposes contradictions which exist in our beliefs about biology and culture, sex and ideology, and women and femininity. By its very presence in society, it sheds light on such questions. Does the source of vast differences between men and women lie in biology or culture and furthermore structure? How are biology and culture defined in society? Are women "naturally female" and men "naturally male" or does culture play a large part in defining femininity and masculinity? What is "natural" or "human nature"? Do they exist or are our beliefs about sexuality based on a false foundation? And what are our ideas about sex really based on?'

Sexuality and gender

Much confusion about sex stems from an inability to distinguish between sexuality and gender. Whilst sexuality categorises people in relation to those they are romantically and sexually attracted to, gender refers to the social and cultural characteristics associated with men and women respectively. We thus tend to think of men as conventionally 'masculine' and women as 'feminine', although these terms are not rigidly defined. Indeed, behaviour and appearance which European societies generally consider to be 'masculine' may well signify femininity in other cultures. Work, rates of pay, clothes, sport, hobbies and a host of other aspects of our everyday lives are intimately affected by gender. These are the constantly changing processes that 'transform males and females into "men" and "women" ' (Vance, 1983).

Whilst the outward appearances of gender can change dramatically even in a single decade, the structured inequality that exists between women and men remains intact. Hence the importance of Rubin's (1975) observation that: 'Far from being an expression of natural differences, exclusive gender identity is the suppression of natural similarities'. In modern-day Western culture, it is the gender system which trains women to be passive and dependent on men, while men are expected to be confident, competent and in control.

Few of us actually live out our lives in these over-simplified roles, and many conflicts and contradictions emerge between the overlapping domains of sexuality and gender. Whilst women and men may share qualities associated with both gender (for example, bossiness, timidity, aggression, sensuality) and sexuality (passion, reticence, lust and desire), their experiences of these may differ considerably.

5.3 SEXUAL PREFERENCES, SEXUAL DESIRES

Numerous myths and prejudices about sex and sexuality are sustained by people's anxiety about talking honestly about their desires, fears and hopes. Recent surveys have shown, for example, that parents often feel embarrassed when talking to their children about sex, preferring sex education to be carried out in schools (see for example Allen, 1987). Glossy magazines with an emphasis on personal relationships still call for a 'new openness' between women and men, and many of the workshops we have run in developing *Learning About AIDS* materials have highlighted the unresolved tensions that can exist in sexual relationships.

Public views, private preferences

In these circumstances, it is hardly surprising that there are major discrepancies between the sexual preferences people express publicly and their private desires. For example, whilst high priority is given to vaginal intercourse in sex education, film and television representations and public discussions of sex, research seems to suggest that, privately, people prefer other things. Recent research by Kahn and Davis (1982), for example, has considered the difference between what people might like or want sexually, and what they actually *do*. Their study of 200 men and 200 women, all of whom defined themselves as heterosexual, revealed a startlingly wide range of disparity between individuals' personal sexual preference, and what they imagined other people preferred. Touching, caressing and manual stimulation, for example, were preferred by most of the women to vaginal penetrative intercourse. Men preferred touching and caressing to 'conventional' intercourse as well. But curiously they thought that women preferred male-on-top intercourse to all other forms of sex! They also thought that other men would prefer male-on-top intercourse.

Other widely held but equally inaccurate views include the assumption that sex between women and men is 'natural', whereas sex between members of the same sex is 'unnatural'. If 'unnatural' is taken in this context to mean statistically unusual, then this is clearly not the case. This attitude oversimplifies the range and variety of human sexual behaviours within and between different social groups. According to the American sexologist Kinsey (1948):

'. . . It is wrong to distinguish between two distinct populations, heterosexual and homosexual. The world is not to be divided into sheep and goats. Not all things are black or all things white . . . Only the human mind invents categories and tries to force facts into separate pigeon-holes. The living world is a continuum in each and every one of its aspects . . . It would encourage clearer thinking on these matters if persons were not characterised as heterosexual or homosexual, but as individuals who have had certain amounts of heterosexual experience and certain amounts of homosexual experience . . .'

In a less often quoted passage, Kinsey observes:

' . . . Biologists and psychologists who have accepted the doctrine that the only natural function of sex is reproduction have simply ignored the existence of sexual activity which is not reproductive. They have assumed that heterosexual responses are a part of an animal's innate, 'instinctive' equipment, and that all other types of sexual activity represent 'perversions' of the 'normal' instincts. Such interpretations are, however, mystical . . .'

In other words, human sexuality encompasses a far wider range of behaviours and identities than is sometimes acknowledged. It is also important to recognise that the same sexual act can take on different meanings depending on who is involved and where it takes place. It may also change its significance according to when it occurs in a person's life. There are no intrinsic meanings associated with particular sexual acts beyond those that are given to them by the context in which they occur. For example, sexual intercourse, whether anal or vaginal, may represent love for one couple, yet express hatred or contempt for another. In this respect, sexuality can never be isolated from its social context.

Many of these ideas are captured sensitively in the writing of the British historian Weeks (1986). He describes sexuality as:

' . . . a transmission belt for a wide variety of needs and desires: for love and anger, tenderness and aggression, intimacy and adventure, romance and predatoriness, pleasure and pain, empathy and power . . . At the same time, the very mobility of sexuality, its chameleon-like ability to take many guises and forms, so that what for one might be a source of warmth and attraction, for another might be one of fear and hate, makes it a particularly sensitive conductor of cultural influences, and hence of social and political divisions'.

Sexual expression and social control

Laws govern every aspect of sex, from the age of consent (currently fixed at 16 for heterosexuals and 21 for gay men) and the circumstances in which sex may or may not take place, to taxation rights, immigration rights, adoption and parenting.

Taxation   Lesbian and gay couples are unable to claim any equivalent to a married man's tax allowance, for example, or a wife's pension on her husband's national insurance. Nor are lesbian or gay spouses guaranteed inheritance rights if their partner dies without making a will.

Immigration   Since lesbians and gay men are unable to marry their partners, the situation often occurs in which a relationship with a non-British national falls foul of immigration law. Whereas in Australia, Holland, Sweden and other countries same-sex couples have equal immigration rights as the rest of the population, such couples cannot claim emotional commitment in order to remain together in the UK. As Crane (1984) has pointed out, many 'gay people have been refused entry or have had to leave Britain despite close emotional ties here.'

Laws like these vary widely around the world, suggesting that there is no readily available or universal consensus about any aspect of sexual behaviour as is immediately apparent if we consider the different ages of consent which apply throughout Europe.

Figure 14: The legal status of homosexuality
European laws regarding minimum age for lawful homosexual relationships between men.

	Legal status of homosexuality
Austria	legal at the age of 18
Belgium	legal at the age of 18 (sexual conduct between two men, both between 18 and 21, is legal, but if one is under 21 and the other over, it is a criminal offence)
Bulgaria	legal at 21
Cyprus	completely illegal for males
Czechoslovakia	legal at 18
Denmark	legal at 15
Eire	completely illegal for males
Finland	legal at 18
France	legal at 15
German Democratic Republic	legal at 18
Federal German Republic	legal at 18
United Kingdom	
England & Wales	legal at 21
Northern Ireland	legal at 21
Scotland	legal at 21
Greece	legal at 17
Holland	legal at 16
Hungary	legal at 10
Iceland	legal at 18
Italy	no special legal restrictions applicable
Luxembourg	legal at 18
Malta	legal at 18
Norway	no special legal restrictions
Portugal	no special legal restrictions
Romania	completely illegal for males
USSR	completely illegal for males
Poland	legal at 15

From Crane, P. (1982) *Gays and the Law,* London, Pluto Press.

Moreover, both sexuality and gender may be manipulated to the purposes of social control and authority. In this context, we should note that, in Britain in 1985, no fewer than 37 men were sent to prison with average sentences of 22 months for having *consensual* sex with other men who were above the heterosexual age of consent, but below that currently set for gay men.

5.4   SEXUAL GROUPS AND SEXUAL IDENTITIES

One of the distinctive characteristics of the modern world is that sexuality is experienced as a fundamental aspect of our nature as human beings. As Rubin (1984) has pointed out:

' . . . Contemporary conflicts over sexual values and erotic conduct have much in common with the religious disputes of earlier centuries. They acquire immense symbolic weight. Disputes over sexual behaviour often become the vehicles for displacing social anxieties, and discharging their attendant emotional intensity. Consequently, sexuality should be treated with special respect in times of great social stress . . . '

In this section we will examine a variety of different kinds of sexuality as well as the implications of these for the formation of particular sexual identities and particular ways of knowing ourselves.

Heterosexuality

Heterosexuality is regarded as the most 'natural', most 'inevitable' and most 'logical' kind of sexual behaviour as well as the least well understood. Rarely defined itself, heterosexuality is the yardstick against which other forms of sexual expression are often judged. In these circumstances, it is easy to take heterosexuality for granted, as if it were self-evident. However, heterosexuality is in fact a complex phenomenon. As Weeks (1986) has put it:

' . . . The term embraces rape as well as loving relationships, coercion as well as choice. It covers a multitude of sexual practices from intercourse in the missionary position to oral and anal intercourse. As a term it obscures differences of age, of institutionalization and even the fantasies of the partners involved . . . '

Heterosexuality is not tied to particular sexual acts, rather it is a statement of the sex of the partners involved in these acts and the relationships between them. A recent survey reported by Veitch and Radford (1987), for example, suggested that one in ten female students at a British university regularly enjoyed anal intercourse — an activity which in some quarters is popularly perceived as the prerogative of gay men. Heterosexuality is also an elastic category since some women and men who consider themselves to be heterosexual (rather than bisexual or lesbian or gay) have also enjoyed same-sex relationships. Heterosexuality's naturalness and inevitability makes the development of a distinctive heterosexual identity difficult, as does women's and men's very different experience of what it is to be heterosexual.

These are important considerations because most people think of themselves as heterosexual in the most casual and unproblematic way. In education about HIV and AIDS, the sheer variety of heterosexuality needs to be stressed, since it relates closely to the many different ways in which women and men can express their feelings and desires.

Tremendous cultural pressures are put on young people in relation to their sexuality, with the expectation that they are not fully adult until they have experienced penetrative vaginal intercourse. Given the high premium that many give to sexual satisfaction in our culture, some sexual experimentation is inevitable. Besides, we all know from our own experience that sexual competence and, more importantly, sexual pleasure is generally only gradually learned and achieved. Although it may seem so in retrospect, sex to begin with rarely involves 'doing what comes naturally'. On the contrary, people discover their sexual potentials and their particular sexual pleasures over a considerable period of time. This may prove difficult to reconcile with the strong social pressures to marry young and start a family. Whilst people are supposed ideally to be sexually confident from an early age, this is by no means necessarily the case, and young women in particular have to overcome the cultural expectations which ensure 'it hasn't been in society's or men's interests for girls to be outspoken about their needs' (*Social Trends,* 1988). As one young woman pointed out in a recent British television programme about AIDS: 'You have to kiss a lot of frogs before you meet your prince.' And, it might be added, if your prince (or princess) disappears, you may have to start kissing frogs again!

Lesbian and gay sexuality

In contrast to heterosexuality which is highly valued socially, morally and legally, lesbian and gay sexuality are still widely regarded as 'abnormal' or 'deviant'.

Since many lesbians and gay men still feel obliged to hide or disguise their sexuality at work or even within their families for fear of rejection, discrimination or even violence, many people are unfortunately ignorant of what it means to grow up lesbian or gay. This type of ignorance can fuel prejudice and superstition. It can also be seen in the efforts that are sometimes made to understand lesbian and gay sexuality in exclusively heterosexual terms, as if all gay men were sexually 'active' or 'passive', for example. In this respect, it seems to matter little that these same distinctions do not always make sense of heterosexual sex.

Similarly, it is often believed that gay male relationships must inevitably involve bodily penetration and anal sex. These beliefs are not only inaccurate and misleading, they also limit our understanding of what it is to be a sexual being. Moreover, by regarding notions of sexual activity and sexual passivity as if they are inherent properties of lesbians and gay men, heterosexual culture is able to sustain powerful biological notions of femininity and masculinity which are ultimately as damaging to men as they are to women.

As a result of their sexuality, lesbians and gay men often experience ridicule, social and moral disapprobation and oppression from early on in their lives. Dominant notions of 'respectable' family life, for example, ensure that many young lesbians and gay men continue to be expelled from their homes by their parents. As one 20-year-old in Trenchard and Warren's recent (1985) study explained: 'They threw me out of the house and didn't speak to me for months. My mother said that she wished that she had had a miscarriage while carrying me.' Another 16-year-old boy described his parents' reaction to the discovery that he was gay thus: 'They nearly dropped dead and couldn't accept it. Now they're worse. They just given me two months to leave home' (Trenchard and Warren, 1985). Unfortunately most families can expect little or no help or support in coming to terms with the fact that their children may be lesbian or gay, and are especially vulnerable to the types of negative myths which abound in the mass media.

As adults, gay men and lesbians are no less subject to prejudice, derision and oppression within education, from 'friends', at work and on the street, and it is in this context that the development of gay and lesbian identities can best be understood. Weeks (1986) has argued that lesbians and gay men have organised their lives in relation to their sexual identities and sexual politics because: 'It was in their sexuality that they felt most powerfully invalidated.' The development of lesbian and gay identities may thus be seen as the outcome of resistance to stereotyped and over-simplified assumptions about gender and sexuality. Whilst being gay is rarely experienced by men as a conscious choice, many lesbians speak of 'choosing' their sexuality. Health educators should recognise that there is no such thing as a single lesbian identity (Kitzinger, 1987).

Bisexuality

Considerable numbers of women and men enjoy sexual relationships with members of both sexes. These relationships vary in number and intensity as much as any others, but given their relative invisibility, bisexuals have not yet found an opportunity to develop a collective identity. There is currently widespread public discomfort about bisexuality as a recent article in *Newsweek* (Gelman *et al*, 1987) entitled 'Bisexuals and AIDS' makes clear. Subtitled 'The Dangers of a Double Life', the article suggests that:

' . . . Male bi's could represent a new dimension in the deadly epidemic. Many doctors consider them among the most likely potential conduits for the spread of AIDS to heterosexuals — who may bed them or, as often happens, marry them, never suspecting that their partners are leading a dangerous double love life . . . '

Behind this sort of anxiety are more profound fears about gay sexuality, and within contemporary debate about AIDS, bisexuals are often identified as a 'bridging group' between the supposedly discrete gay and heterosexual populations. It is important to recognise that this type of explanation is rooted in a kind of epidemiology which represents the social world as a series of separate and self-contained groups.

It is not always helpful to think of bisexuality as a distinct form of sexuality or of bisexuals as distinct types of women and men, for bisexuality serves to reveal the general inadequacy of the sexual categories we have already referred to. Nevertheless, some people may identify themselves as bisexual in a similar manner to lesbians and gay men, feeling themselves also to be marginalised by the dominant view that everyone either is, or should be, compulsorily heterosexual.

New sexual groupings, new sexual identities

The new sexual groupings that exist in the Western world stand for a more open and democratic approach to the inevitable diversity of sexual desire. They are concrete evidence of the wide range of ways in which people can live together and enjoy sexual partnerships. It is in this sense that health educators may find it most helpful to think about the different sexual groups which make up our society, and contribute so much to the richness and diversity of its culture. While there could no more be a single 'gay community' than there could be a single 'heterosexual community', it is important to be aware of the possibilities that lesbian and gay culture offer, by offering opportunities for the kind of self-esteem that many other people can take for granted in the course of growing up. Ultimately, the diversity of human sexuality simply cannot be denied.

References

Allen, I. (1987) *Education in Sex and Personal Relationships,* London, Policy Studies Institute.

Crane, P. (1982) *Gays and the Law,* London, Pluto Press.

Ettorre, E.M. (1980) *Lesbians, Women and Society,* London, Routledge & Kegan Paul.

Gelman, D. *et al* (1987) Bisexuals and AIDS: the dangers of a double life, *Newsweek,* 13 July.

Herzlich, C. & Pierret, J. (1986) Illness: from causes to meaning, in C. Currer & M. Stacey (eds), *Concepts of Health, Illness and Disease: A Comparative Perspective,* Leamington Spa, Berg.

Kahn, S. & Davis, J. (1982) *The Kahn Report on Sexual Preferences.* New York, Avon Books.

Kinsey, A.C. *et al* (1948) *Sexual Behaviour in the Human Male.* Philadelphia.

Kitzinger, C. (1987) *The Social Construction of Lesbianism,* Beverly Hills, Sage.

Plummer, K. (1986) Sexual diversity: a sociological perspective, in K. Howells (ed) *The Psychology of Sexual Diversity,* Oxford, Blackwell.

Rubin, G. (1975) The traffic in women: notes on the 'political economy' of sex, in R. R. Reiter (ed) *Towards an Anthropology of Women,* New York, Monthly Review Press.

Rubin, G. (1984) Thinking sex: notes for a radical theory of the politics of sexuality, in C. Vance (ed) *Pleasure and Danger: Exploring Female Sexuality,* London, Routledge & Kegan Paul.

Social Trends (1988) 18th ed, Government Central Statistical Office, London.

Trenchard, L. & Warren, H. (1985) *Something to Tell You.* London Gay Teenage Group, London.

Vance, C. (1983) Gender systems, ideology and sex research, in A. Snitow (ed) *Desire: the politics of sexuality,* London, Virago.

Veitch, A. & Radford, T. (1987) Students switch to less casual sex, *Guardian,* 28 August.

Weeks, J. (1986) *Sexuality,* London, Tavistock.

6.   Safer sex

Given that the most common mode of HIV transmission worldwide involves unprotected sexual intercourse with an infected person (Adler, 1987), education about safer sex is a key issue in health education about HIV infection and AIDS. In this section, we will discuss what safer sex is and describe some of the sexual options open to women and men.

It is inaccurate to suggest that everyone is at equal risk of HIV infection. Whilst anyone who has unprotected sex with another person may potentially be at risk (in the sense that the other person might be infected and capable of passing the infection on), some social groups are presently far more vulnerable than others because the distribution of HIV infection throughout the population is uneven.

Neither is it very helpful to suggest that for some social groups the risk of HIV infection is negligible or non-existent. The relationship between sexual identity and sexual behaviour is not clear cut, and safer sex education will need to provide opportunities for people to identify their own risks, not as members of supposedly 'at risk' or 'not at risk' groups, but as individuals whose present repertoire of sexual behaviour may or may not pose a threat to their own health and that of others.

It is important to recognise that whilst the present incidence of AIDS amongst particular groups in Britain tells us much about past patterns of infection, it tells us little about future changes in these. It is therefore crucial to help people identify ways in which they can minimise their own risk of infection and that of others.

6.1   WHAT IS SAFER SEX

What is safer sex, and what is it that education about safer sex tries to achieve? Put succinctly, the aim of safer sex education is to encourage forms of sexual expression in which the risk of HIV transmission is minimised. Given what is known about HIV's modes of transmission (see Section 2.5), safer sex aims to ensure that semen, blood and cervical and vaginal secretions do not pass from one person to another: via the vagina, via the rectum, via breaks in the skin or via damage to the gums and the lining of the mouth.

There are many ways in which safer sexual activity can take place, but ultimately it will be for individuals and their sexual partners to decide what is most pleasurable and acceptable. Education about safer sex is therefore likely to involve:

a) helping people assess possible risks of HIV infection by considering its modes of transmission.

b) helping people identify the most acceptable safer sexual options for themselves and their partner(s).
c) supporting people if they decide that changes need to be made to their sexual behaviour.

To be successful, education about safer sex should proceed from trust rather than fear. It should also be underpinned by a respect for the many ways in which consensual sexual relationships can take place, rather than from a desire to promote one or more of these above others. Safer sex education should aim to help people protect themselves and their partners from HIV infection, rather than to pass judgement on particular kinds of sexual behaviour. People need support and respect if they are to identify *for themselves, and with others,* safer ways of expressing themselves sexually. In the midst of uncertainty and anxiety, education about safer sex is therefore a way of helping people make safer and more responsible decisions.

The first information about safer sex appeared in the United States, produced by and for gay men (Altman, 1986). Subsequently, equivalent material was produced in Britain by voluntary sector such as the Terrence Higgins Trust. The work of organisations such as this has been supported by District Health Authorities, Local Authorities and organisations such as the Family Planning Association (FPA).

Much of the early literature on safer sex emphasised collective and community responsibility. An influential booklet prepared by and for gay men in 1983 argued: 'Since we are a community, taking responsibility for our *own* health during sex ultimately requires that we protect our *partner's* health as well as our own' (Berkowitz & Callen, 1983). The writers went on to emphasize, 'When you are deciding what sexual acts will take place, you must not only ask: "Will this pose a health risk to me?" but also, "Will this pose a health risk to my partner?" '

At a time when the origins and causes of AIDS were poorly understood, it is perhaps not surprising that there were a number of tensions and contradictions in this early literature. Some of these concerned the extent to which the *number of sexual partners,* as opposed to the *nature of the sexual acts* that takes place between them, was critical in determining the risk of infection. The second, related to distinctions between *high-risk groups* and *high-risk behaviours.*

From early on in the epidemic it was believed that the more sexual partners individuals had, the greater would be the risk of them acquiring HIV infection. The evidence to support such a claim came originally from North American case-control epidemiological studies of gay men carried out early in the epidemic — a context in which safer sex as we now know it was rarely practised (see, for example, Goedert *et al,* 1984). In many of these studies, the number of sexual partners a person had had was often identified as a good predictor of whether or not they had HIV infection or AIDS — a finding which is not at all surprising in the context of unprotected sex. It seemed sensible therefore to recommend that people cut down their number of sexual partners in order to reduce the risk.

Now that more has been learned about the origins of AIDS and HIV's very specific modes of transmission, some health educators have found it useful to qualify the advice they give. Whilst having many sexual partners may increase the chance of *encountering* someone with HIV infection, whether or not it increases the chances of *acquiring* the infection depends on the kinds of sexual acts that take place between the individuals concerned. So long as the blood, semen, cervical and vaginal secretions of one person do not pass to another, transmission can not take place. By adopting safer sexual practices, and by *adhering to them in every sexual encounter,* it is therefore possible (although some would say morally undesirable) for someone to have sex with many partners and significantly reduce the risk of infection. This risk can, of course, be further reduced by limiting the number of sexual partners, or indeed by abstaining from all forms of sex. Ultimately it must be for individuals and their partners to decide what for them constitutes an acceptable degree of risk. It is the responsibility of health educators to provide opportunities for this kind of risk assessment to take place.

Whilst it first seemed sensible to talk about high- and low-risk groups, on the assumption that gay men, injecting drug users, heterosexuals and so on formed homogeneous, discrete and easily identifiable communities, it has subsequently been recognised that not everyone in one of these high-risk groups participates in high-risk sexual activity. Neither is it necessarily the case that those who practice high-risk behaviour are members of high risk-groups. In consequence, as Shernoff (1987) has observed, many health educators now talk about high- and low-risk behaviours rather than high- and low-risk groups.

However, this emphasis on behaviour produces certain difficulties of its own. For just as the notion of high-risk groups persuaded many people that they did not have to think about HIV at all, so the notion of risky behaviours can lead some, equally misleadingly, to the view that safer sex simply means avoiding certain sexual acts, especially anal intercourse. Health educators should encourage people to assess realistically the risks which may accompany *any* form of sexual contact that permits the transmission of HIV.

6.2 THE ISSUE OF LANGUAGE

Anxiety about sex and the absence of a common vocabulary in which to discuss it poses a particular problem, and has led some health educators to avoid the topic altogether. Others have found it difficult to be explicit about safer sexual options, and have couched their descriptions of safer sex in obscure scientific terminology, or in indirect and euphemistic language. Many early safer sex health education responses talked extensively, for example, about the importance of 'not exchanging body fluids' during sex. It is best to avoid using ambiguous phrases like these.

Similar difficulties can arise when health educators inadvertently use phrases such as 'sexual intercourse', 'making love' and 'heavy petting' without having first clarified what they mean by them and without having found out what others understand by them.

Other problems can arise if sex is talked about too explicitly without having first checked out with a group what is acceptable. In health education about safer sex, it is best therefore to identify early on the kind of language people feel most comfortable with.

6.3   SAFER SEXUAL OPTIONS

Some of the more talked about safer sexual options include celibacy, chastity, monogamy and the use of condoms. A variety of other practices are less talked about, either as a result of anxiety, or as a result of the tendency to equate sex with bodily penetration.

People wanting to adopt safer sex as a permanent way of life, rather than as an occasional practice, may also need to develop particular social skills, especially when others around them may be less aware of the need to take precautions against HIV. Issues to do with power, control, honesty and responsibility also arise here. Health educators are likely to have an increasingly important role in helping others cope with these.

Celibacy and chastity

Throughout history, a number of groups and individuals have renounced sexual behaviour altogether, either for spiritual or secular reasons. This kind of behaviour is usually referred to as chastity or celibacy (which technically means the unmarried state).

Among adults, complete celibacy (where all sexual behaviour is renounced) is a rare response to AIDS, and may sometimes be associated with sexual anxieties which pre-date AIDS but which are stimulated by fears about it. Whilst it is important to respect the reasons why someone may decide to abstain from sex, an unreasonable fear of HIV infection is perhaps not the best of reasons for reaching such a decision. Moreover, those who take up celibacy in response to AIDS do not automatically find the experience reassuring (Miller, 1986). Their anxieties and fears concerning AIDS and/or sexuality may remain a source of recurring tension. This may explain why some who initially resort to celibacy as a response to AIDS, periodically revert to extremely unsafe sexual practices, in a recurring 'diet/binge' pattern (Shernoff, 1987).

Monogamy

Like celibacy, the meaning of monogamy is not necessarily self-evident. For some, monogamy means sexual fidelity to one partner for life. For others, monogamy means a series of such relationships. If a couple have been entirely monogamous since before the emergence of HIV, if neither of them is a haemophiliac, if neither has received a blood transfusion, and if neither has shared equipment in connection with injecting drug use, then it is extremely unlikely that they will be at risk of HIV infection. This situation is likely to prevail until one or both partners has unprotected sex with another person, or otherwise puts themselves at risk.

However, for those just beginning a sexual relationship, it is possible that one or both partners may have been infected through their previous sexual encounters. In this situation, monogamy will not provide protection against HIV. It is therefore essential for individuals to be honest about their sexual histories before beginning a new sexual relationship. If worried, they should seek professional advice about whether or not it would be useful to have an HIV antibody test.

It is important to recognise that it is dangerous to counsel monogamy as an end in itself to those who have been at risk of infection. In these circumstances, it would be more appropriate to explore with individuals the desirability of an HIV test and the need to adopt safer sexual practices.

Condoms

Since the early 1980s, condoms have played a central role in discussions about safer sex. If they are effectively used, condoms can reduce the risk of transmitting HIV during penetrative sexual intercourse and oral sex. They are therefore an important way of making sex safer. They also protect against most other sexually transmitted diseases. As a form of contraception they have a failure rate of between 5–15%. Much of this can be put down to incorrect use, and health educators have a role to play in advising people how to use them correctly.

Using condoms   A man who has not used condoms will need to practise with them before having penetrative intercourse of any kind. Uncircumcised men will need to retract the foreskin first, before rolling the condom down the full length of the penis. The last centimetre of the closed end should be squeezed when putting the condom on to expel trapped air and make space for the semen. The Health Education Authority's leaflet *Your Guide to Safer Sex and the Condom* provides further guidance on this. Condoms should be used with a water-based lubricant. Hand-creams, body oils and vaseline should never be used as lubricants since they rot they material from which condoms are made. The penis should always be withdrawn from the partner after ejaculation and before the erection has subsided. The visible part of the condom should be held firmly in place at the base of the penis as withdrawal takes place in order to ensure that the condom does not stay inside the partner.

Choosing condoms   There are many different kinds of condoms available from chemists and a growing range of other stores (Figure 15). Some are already lubricated, some contain a spermicidal agent called Nonoxynol 9 which has been shown in laboratory conditions to be effective against HIV (Hicks *et al*, 1985), and some are thicker than others, having been designed, so their manufacturers claim, with safer sex in mind.

Figure 15: Survey of condoms

Brand	Pence per condom [1]	Country of manufacture	Kitemarked	Colour	Surface	Shape	Teat ended
Aegis Anti-VD	[3]	not stated	no	beige	smooth	plain [4]	yes
Aegis Big Boy [7]	35	W Germany	no	beige	smooth	plain	no
Aegis Snugfit [7]	30	W Germany	no	beige	smooth	plain	no
Blausiegel Hauch-dunn Extra [7]	23	W Germany	no	beige	smooth	plain	yes
Blausiegel Koralle [7]	83	W Germany	no	pink	rough	plain	yes
Duet Supersafe Fully Shaped	28	W Germany	no	beige	smooth	contoured	yes
Duet Supersafe Ribbed	32	W Germany	no	beige	ribbed	contoured	yes
Duet Supersafe Studded	32	W Germany	no	beige	studded	plain	yes
Duet Supersafe Ultra Thin	30	W Germany	no	beige	smooth	plain	yes
Durex Arouser	26	UK	yes	pink	ribbed	plain	yes
Durex Black Shadow	26	UK	yes	black	smooth	plain	yes
Durex Elite	26	UK	yes	beige	smooth	plain	yes
Durex Fetherlite	21	UK	yes	pink	smooth	plain	yes
Durex Fiesta	25	UK	yes	pink, blue, green, black	smooth	plain	yes
Durex Gold	29	UK	yes	gold	smooth	plain	no
Durex Gossamer [9]	22	UK	yes	beige	smooth	plain	yes
Durex Nu-form Extra Safe	22	UK	yes	pink	smooth	contoured	yes
Erotim Banana Hit [7]	70	W Germany	no	pink	smooth	plain	yes
Forget-Me-Not [10]	16	UK	yes	beige	smooth	plain	yes
Fulex Rony Wrinkle	42	Taiwan	no	pink, green and violet	ribbed	contoured	yes
Gold Knight	10	Korea	no	beige	smooth	contoured	yes
HT Special [7]	58	W Germany	no	beige	smooth	plain	yes
Jiffi Gold	25	not stated	no	beige	smooth	contoured	yes
Knight Barrier	16	Korea	no	beige	smooth	plain	yes
Lambutt Safetex [13]	15	UK	yes	beige	smooth	plain	yes
Lambutt Tru-Shape [13]	18	UK	yes	pink	smooth	contoured	yes
Lifestyles Nuda	17	USA	yes	beige	smooth	plain	yes
Lifestyles Stimula	18	USA	no	beige	ribbed	contoured	yes
Mentor	[14]	USA	no	beige	smooth	plain	yes
Personal Extra Thin [7] [15]	29	Italy	no	beige	smooth	plain	yes
Premex Coral Superfine Dry [16]	19	UK	no	pink	smooth	plain	yes
Prime [17]	33	USA	no	beige	smooth	contoured	yes
Red Stripe [18]	33	Japan	no	beige	smooth	plain	no
Skin Less Skin	27	Japan	no	pink and green	smooth	plain	yes
Sweet Rider	42	USA	no	beige	studded	contoured	yes

From *Self-Health*, September 1987.
This survey was completed before the launch in 1987 of *Lifestyles Extra* and the *Mates* range of condoms.
Key to ratings: the more blobs the better.

Dressing [2]	Instructions	Thickness (mm)	Freedom from holes	Strength
P	[5]	0.21	fail	[6]
P	[5]	0.06	pass	●●
L	●●	0.05	pass	●●
L	●●●	0.06	pass	●●
L	[5]	0.05	[20]	●●
SL	●●●	0.06	pass	●●
SL	●●●	0.06	fail	●●
SL	●●●	0.06	fail	●●
SL	●●●	0.05	pass	●●
L	●●	0.06	pass	●●
L	●●	0.05	pass	●●
SLN	●●●●	0.05	pass	●●
L	●●[8]	0.05	pass	●●
L	●●	0.05	pass	●●
SLN	●●	0.05	pass	●●
L	●●[8]	0.05	pass	●●
SLN	●●●[8]	0.05	pass	●●
S	[5]	0.06	pass	●●
L	●●●	0.06	pass	●●
L	●●	0.04	pass	●
L	●●●●	0.05	pass	●●
L	●●●	0.09	pass	●●●●
SLN	●●●●	0.05	pass	●●
L[11]	[12]	0.07	pass	●●
L	●●●	0.06	pass	●●
L	●●●	0.06	pass	●●
L	●●●	0.05	pass	●●
L	●●●	0.06	pass	●●
L	●●●	0.05	pass	●●
L	[5]	0.06	pass	●●
P	●	0.05	pass	●●
SLN	●●●●	0.07	pass	●●
L	●●	0.06	pass	●●
L	●[19]	0.03	pass	●
L	●●	0.06	fail	●●

Condoms which failed our tests are printed in white on black

[1] Typical selling prices based on packets of 10 or 12 or smaller packs where these are not available

[2] L = lubricant; SL = spermicidal lubricant; SLN = spermicidal lubricant with nonoxynol-9; P = powder; S = scented

[3] Now discontinued

[4] With additional sac for scrotum

[5] Instructions were missing from some of our packets. Where they existed they merited ●●

[6] There were too many holes in this condom for us to be able to complete our strength tests

[7] Also available by mail order from Aegis Products, Roman Way, Coleshill, Birmingham B46 1RL

[8] Larger packets carried better instructions

[9] Also distributed by family planning clinics under the Atlas name

[10] Also sold with spermicidal pessaries as Two's Company. Both are available by mail order from Family Planning Sales, 28 Kelburne Road, Cowley, Oxford OX4 3SZ

[11] The manufacturers tell us this will have a spermicidal lubricant containing nonoxynol-9 from Septmber 1988

[12] Instructions were missing from some of our packets. Where they existed, they merited ●●●

[13] Also available by mail order from Lamberts (Dalston) Ltd, PO Box 93, Luton LU1 5BW.

[14] Costs over £1 in the United States. The American manufacturers have not yet set a date for expanding to the UK

[15] Also sold as Personal Naturale

[16] Also available by mail order from Premier Laboratories Ltd, 11 Black Lion Street, Brighton BN1 1PJ

[17] Also available by mail order from The Sentry Box, 54 Cornigh House, Royal Road, Kennington Park, London SE17 3NT

[18] Also available by mail order from 'Red Stripe', Britannia House, Hammersmith, London W5 0LF

[19] The manufacturers tell us they now plan to include instructions

[20] Condom passed the hole test, but had more than the allowable number of other manufacturing defects.

Since the data in Figure 15 were published, Warner Lambert have introduced a new condom called 'Lifestyles – Extra' and Virgin Healthcare have brought out a range of condoms under the brand-name 'Mates'.

To equate safer sex with condom use is limiting as it ignores women's and men's different feelings about penetrative intercourse. Given the many ways in which people can express themselves sexually, health education which does not move beyond condom use may also leave many questions unanswered.

Other safer sexual options

As was discussed earlier, there are many ways in which people can express themselves sexually. Only a few of these involve bodily penetration, and only some involve orgasm. Other very pleasurable kinds of sexual behaviour include kissing, touching, holding, hugging, nibbling, rubbing, stroking and caressing. Some involve individuals stimulating their own genitals or those of their partner. Provided that none of these behaviours allows semen, blood, cervical or vaginal secretions to enter another person, through the rectum, vagina or cuts and abrasions on the skin or in the mouth, they can be regarded as safer sexual practices.

It is important for health educators to respect the many ways in which consensual sexual activity can take place. There are many sexual practices which are sometimes regarded as unusual, or even extreme, involving sexual role-play, cross-dressing or physical restraint: many of these can be free from any risk of HIV transmission.

Health educators may find that unless they take care to structure their work on safer sex carefully, so as to ensure that a discussion of these alternative forms of sexual expression takes place, some groups may be unwilling to talk about them, perhaps through embarrassment or perhaps because of a tendency to equate sex only with bodily penetration and orgasm.

Dildoes and other sex toys

Dildoes and other sex toys are sometimes used by men and women as a means of gaining sexual pleasure. Common sense and normal standards of hygiene suggest that sex toys should be properly cleaned after use, but the advent of HIV infection suggests that special care needs to be taken in certain circumstances. It is inadvisable for people at risk of HIV infection to share toys. Disinfection between use in a solution of one part bleach to ten parts of water is also to be recommended. As in the case of all sexual relationships, people should try to be honest with themselves and with their partners when using toys. They should try to avoid acting against their own wishes or those of others.

Other sexual practices

Early safer sex literature often listed large numbers of specific sexual acts, grouped together according to criteria of safety or risk of HIV transmission.

This meant that sexual behaviours which were enjoyed by a small minority received as much attention as more common sexual practices.

If any kind of sexual behaviour allows blood, semen or vaginal and cervical secretions to enter the body of another person, there will be a risk of transmission if one of the partners has HIV infection. While HIV has not been shown to be transmitted via faeces, there are sound health reasons of a more general kind to suggest that 'scat' (sex involving defecation) and 'rimming' (mouth-to-anus contact) are best avoided. Similar considerations apply to 'watersports' (sex involving urine). 'Fisting' which involves the insertion of the hand or forearm into the vagina or rectum of another person, has been known to cause severe internal injuries with consequent loss of blood, and rectal or vaginal 'fingering' can also lead to bleeding. Unless a barrier such as a rubber glove or rubber finger stall is involved, these activities may carry a substantial risk if one of the parties involved has HIV infection.

In responding to questions about sexual practices other than these, it is a good idea for health educators to use their knowledge about the ways in which HIV *is* and *is not* transmitted to work out the risks concerned with those asking the question.

6.4 SAFER SEX EDUCATION AND PARTICULAR GROUPS

While it is possible to identify a general set of principles that should inform all discussion about safer sex, if this kind of education is to be successful, it must also speak directly to the needs of different groups of people.

Heterosexual women

Richardson (1986) has recently pointed out that communication is vital to safer sex — 'it is important that you say what you want, and negotiate what you can do together.' Given the nature of many male–female relationships, in which women may be expected to comply with their partners' sexual wishes regardless of what they themselves want, this may be a difficult goal to achieve.

Some women may find themselves in a difficult situation if they carry condoms, being regarded as 'promiscuous' or 'a slag' by men. This demonstrates a double standard at work, since men often want women to be available for sex, but not prepared, or even necessarily willing.

Health education about HIV infection and AIDS which emphasises condom use as a means of making penetrative sex safer may also reinforce the tendency to understand women's sexuality in exclusively male terms. There are major differences between women's and men's experience of penetrative sex, and to equate safer sex with condom use may fail to tackle the issue of sexual fulfilment for women in some heterosexual relationships.

Health educators will find it useful to consider the most effective strategies by which to empower heterosexual women in their negotiations with heterosexual men about safer sex. Opportunities may need to be provided for heterosexual women to share their experiences with one another and to identify ways in which they can express their needs more assertively in sexual relationships.

Complex issues can arise when a woman who has been practising safer sex wishes to become pregnant and at the same time wants to be sure that she does not put herself at risk of HIV infection. There are no simple answers to this particular dilemma, but she should carefully assess with her partner (and perhaps with her doctor) whether or not an HIV antibody test would be appropriate (see Section 3.3).

Lesbians

Much of the literature on safer sex has been designed to meet the needs of gay men and heterosexual women and men. So far little has been produced for or by lesbians. This is particularly worrying since some lesbians may be at risk of HIV infection either through their sexual relationships with men or through those with other women.

This general lack of information may relate to the social marginalisation of lesbians in society, but it also serves to reinforce their apparent invisibility (Faderman, 1981). It has also led some lesbians to identify themselves as a 'low risk' group so far as HIV transmission is concerned. However, the fact that few lesbians have so far been directly affected by AIDS is no cause for complacency.

There is no such thing as a single lesbian lifestyle, and some lesbians may be involved, willingly or not, in sexual relationships with men. Others may have direct sexual contact with semen for a wide variety of social and economic reasons, including prostitution (Nestle, 1987). Self-insemination can also pose a risk if the donor has HIV infection.

There are as yet few firm statistics on the subject of woman-to-woman transmission, although a number of individual cases have now been documented (Monzon & Capellan, 1987; Greenhouse, 1987). Given what is known about the ways in which HIV is transmitted, there is no reason to assume, as perhaps some lesbians do, that lesbianism in itself offers any guarantee against infection (Hart, 1986). As Patton and Kelly (1987), have pointed out, 'Risk comes from what you do, not how you label yourself.' The notion that lesbian sex is intrinsically safe is potentially misleading and therefore dangerous.

At the same time, health educators should be aware that lesbians have a long cultural history of talking about sex and sharing difficult or painful emotional experiences. Their involvement in the Women's Movement and in aspects of collective health-care provision, including Well Woman Centres and Women's Reproductive Rights groups, strongly suggests that safer sex education among lesbians can call upon a deep tradition of mutual respect and co-operation in matters to do with health and sexuality.

Gay men

Gay men remain more vulnerable to HIV than any other group in Britain because the virus first entered their communities long before its effects and symptoms became apparent. As a result, many gay men have practised safer sex for years, and have much to teach health educators and the rest of the population.

Gay men grow up in a culture which almost invariably denies the validity of their sexual feelings and behaviour. In this context, Goldstein (1983) has observed that heterosexuals 'have no comparable experience, though it may seem so in memory. They are never called upon to deny desire, only to defer its consummation.'

It is therefore particularly important not to create the impression that gay sex is, in itself, dangerous, unhealthy or unsafe. Instead, in their work with gay men as with other groups, health educators should aim 'to make good sex better, by making it safer, rather than make safe sex seem boring, complicated, or something only prudes and wimps are interested in' (Carr, 1985).

Health educators should also avoid an over-emphasis on condom use in their work with gay men, as education about the wide range of safer sexual alternatives will be important. They should also recognise that gay men are likely to be as aware of the risk of possibly transmitting HIV to a sexual partner as much as the risk of contracting it. In this respect, AIDS awareness among gay men is markedly different to AIDS awareness in other groups.

Heterosexual men

For many heterosexual men, sexual expression is firmly linked to penetrative vaginal intercourse. Indeed, there is often a tendency for other forms of sexual behaviour to be seen as foreplay or a substitute for this. In the short term, therefore, safer sex education emphasising condom use is likely to be very important. In the medium to long term, however, it will be important to explore other safer sexual options. A discussion of these can be linked to an exploration of women's needs within heterosexual relationships.

Cultural stereotypes which suggest that 'real men' should be strong and silent make it difficult for many heterosexual men to discuss their sexual and erotic feelings sensitively with one another. Health educators can provide safe opportunities for this to take place. They may find it especially important to challenge competitive notions of sexual prowess, especially when these lead to behaviour which puts women, and men themselves, at risk of HIV.

Bisexuals

Bisexuality is probably more common than many people realise, and the advent of AIDS has focused attention on bisexual men, in the belief that they may form a bridge between gay men and the heterosexual population. Two unrelated sets of issues frequently become confused. The first of these concerns the fact that men with HIV infection may transmit the virus to either women or men via unprotected sex, regardless of whether they consider themselves to be gay, heterosexual or bisexual. The second relates to the fact that HIV infection has been present amongst heterosexuals for as long as it has been amongst gay men. Health education needs to address both of these issues if the needs of bisexual men are to be met and unhelpful prejudices challenged.

The educational needs of bisexual women has been even more overlooked than those of lesbians. Safer sex education for male and female bisexuals has to proceed from an understanding of the ways in which they are frequently rejected both by heterosexuals *and* by lesbians and gay men. They are frequently portrayed as the most dangerous group in society, but may be amongst those most vulnerable to HIV infection. Ill-informed prejudice against bisexuals makes it harder for the individuals concerned to be open and honest about their sexual behaviour.

Young people

Young people have often been identified as a group with special needs within the context of safer sex education. It is often suggested that they are more irresponsible than adults in matters to do with sex. However, safer sex education may stand more chance of success amongst those whose sexual behaviour is less clearly fixed than amongst those with well-established preferences and patterns of behaviour.

The Chair of the American College Health Association has recently pointed out that, contrary to popular belief, adults cannot easily change the sexual behaviour of adolescents (Keeling, cited in Helquist, 1987). Because many young people have a strong sense of their immediate peer group, it may be at this level that safer sex education is likely to be most effective. For this reason, it is especially important that they are encouraged to participate in safer sex education as an ordinary part of social experience. Health educators will therefore have a vital role to play in promoting a positive safer sex culture amongst young people through the work they undertake with schools as well as through that with adults who come into contact with young people.

There is some evidence to suggest that as long as safer sex education begins early enough there is every reason to suggest that young people will be receptive to the issues involved. For example, a survey commissioned by the DHSS recently found that, whereas only one in five of sexually active 22–34-year-olds had used a condom in their last sexual encounter and only one in four of sexually active 18–21-year-olds had done the same, almost half (47%) 16–17-year-olds had done so (DHSS, 1987).

In planning safer sex education with young people, health educators will need to give special consideration to the situation of lesbian and gay teenagers at a time when they can expect little support at home or at school, and when their social isolation may make them highly vulnerable to anxiety, depression and possibly unsafe sex.

References

Adler, M. (1987) *The ABC of AIDS*, London, British Medical Journal Publications.
Altman, D. (1986) *AIDS and the New Puritanism*, London, Pluto Press.
Berkowitz, R. & Callen, M. (1983) *How to Have Sex in an Epidemic*, New York, News from the Front   Publications.
Carr, A. (1985) Safe sex: can you keep it up? *Mister*, 51.
DHSS (1987) *AIDS: Monitoring Response to the Public Education Campaign February 1986– February 1987*, London, HMSO.
Faderman, L. (1981) *Surpassing the Love of Men: Romantic Friendship and Love Between Women from the Renaissance to the Present*, London, Junction Books.
Goedert, J. *et al* (1984) Determinants of retrovirus (HTLV-III) antibody and immunodeficiency conditions in homosexual men, *Lancet*, **ii**, p 711.
Goldstein, R. (1983) Heartsick: fear and loving in gay community, *Village Voice*, **27, 26**, 28 June.
Greenhouse, P. (1987) Female to female transmission of HIV, *Lancet*, **ii**, p 401-2.
Hart, V. (1986) Lesbians and AIDS, *Gossip*, **2**, p 91.
Helquist, M. (1987) Heterosexuals and AIDS: report from Atlanta, *Focus*, **2, 5**, p 3.
Hicks, D. *et al* (1985) Inactivation of HTLV-III/LAV infected cultures of normal human lymphocytes by Nonoxynol 9 in vitro, *Lancet*, **ii**, p 1422.
Miller, D. (1986) The worried well, in *The Management of AIDS Patients*, Basingstoke, Macmillan.
Monzon, O. & Capellan, J. (1987) Female to female transmission of HIV, *Lancet*, **ii**, pp 40-1.
Nestle, J. (1987) Lesbians and prostitutes: a historical sisterhood, in F. Delacost and P. Alexander (eds) *Sex Work: writings by women in the sex industry*. San Francisco, Clies Press.
Patton, C. & Kelly, J. (1987) *Making It: A Woman's Guide to Sex in the Age of AIDS*, New York, Firebrand Books.
Richardson, D. (1987) *Women and the AIDS Crisis*, London, Pandora Press.
Shernoff, M. (1987) Integrating AIDS prevention into clinical practice, *Focus*, **3, 1**, p 1.

7.   Injecting drug use and HIV infection

One of the main ways in which HIV can be transmitted is through direct blood-to-blood contact. This mode of transmission was identified after AIDS had been diagnosed in three groups of people that are likely to come into contact with the blood or blood products of others — haemophiliacs, the recipients of blood transfusions and injecting drug users.

HIV can be transmitted via the exchange of blood that takes place when needles and syringes are shared. Indeed, infection can spread very rapidly this way. In Edinburgh, for example, retrospective testing of stored blood samples for HIV antibodies suggests that the virus was first introduced into the city's injecting drug population around August 1983. By March 1985, however, half of a sample of 150 injecting drug users tested for HIV antibodies had positive results (Robertson, 1987). In New York City, 33% of reported cases of AIDS in 1986 involved injecting drug use, and similar statistics pertain to many other North American cities (Robertson, 1987). Some of those who inject drugs may of course be at risk of HIV infection in other ways if they have unsafe sex with an infected partner. Injecting drug use therefore creates a challenging set of dilemmas for health education about HIV infection and AIDS.

The emphasis in this chapter will be on examining those issues to do with drugs and drug use that are most closely linked to HIV infection and AIDS. Health educators wishing to explore a wider set of concerns than these may find the additional resources identified in Appendix B helpful.

7.1   TERMS AND TERMINOLOGY

In this book, the phase 'injecting drug user' rather than 'intravenous drug user' is deliberately used. Because the latter term implies quite erroneously that injecting drug use takes place only through the veins, we have used a more comprehensive term which covers drug practices such as subcutaneous injection (injection beneath the skin), which some injecting drug users may use as an alternative to intravenous injection.

The term 'drug use' is also used in preference to either 'drug misuse' or 'drug abuse'. Both of the latter terms imply that drug use is either harmful or socially unacceptable. This may be one way of evaluating the acts involved, but in our view, the term 'drug use' is less moralistic. Moreover, people who take drugs usually refer to themselves as drug users rather than drug misusers or drug abusers. We have similarly avoided the use of terms such as 'addict' and 'addiction' because these imply that injecting drug use leads inevitably to drug dependency, with serious effects on the individual and society. A growing body of research shows that this is not necessarily the case (see McGachy, 1985; Pearson, 1987a; ISDD, 1987).

Health educators may also find it helpful to know some of the street terms relating to injecting drug use (Figures 16 and 17). These change rapidly, however, according to fashion, and there are also regional and cultural variations in their use. In the light of this, many workers in the field feel it is more appropriate for clinical terms to be used with clients in order to avoid any misunderstandings that may arise. For instance, between 1978 and 1982 when heroin use and availability increased, it was reported that many young users did not realise that smack or skag was in fact heroin and subsequently made choices based on inaccurate information.

Figure 16: Street terms for some common injectable drugs

Clinical/generic terms	*Street terms*
Amphetamines and Amphetamine-like stimulants	
Amphetamines in general	Uppers, Jolly Beans
Dexedrine (Dexamphetamine)	Dexies (occasionally Dixies), Yellows
Benzedrine (L-amphetamine)	Bennies
Amphetamine Sulphate	Speed, Whizz
Drinamyl (later Durophet-M; amphetamine and dexamphetamine)	Blues or Purple Hearts
Ritalin (Methylphenidate)	
Tenuate Dospan (Diethylpropion)	Tombstone
Opiates	
(i) *Substances derived from the opium poppy*	
Opium, Morphine, Codeine, Heroin and Diacetylmorphine)	Horse smack, Skag, H, Harry, Gear
(ii) *Synthetic opiates*	
Pethidine	
Methadone (Physeptone)	Meth/Phy
Diconal (dipipanone and cyclizine)	Dike
DF118 (Dihydrocodeine)	DF's
Fortral (Pentazocine)	
Temgesic (Buprenorphine)	Temmies

Barbiturates

Barbiturates in general	Barbs, Downers
Phenobarbitone	Barbs
Tuinal (Quinalbarbitone and Amylobarbitone)	Tueys, Traffic Lights
Nembutal (Pentobarbitone)	Yellows, Nembies, Downers, Sleepers
Seconal (Quinalbarbitone)	Reds, Sekkies
Sodium Amytal (Amylobarbitone)	
Pentothal/Intraval (Thiopentone)	

Cocaine

Cocaine hydrochloride	Charlie, Snow, Toot, Lady, Girl, Coke, Crack
Cocaine and Opiates 'doubled up'	Speedball

Figure 17: Street terms for some common injecting practices

Shooting Galleries	Places, especially in the US, where an injecting drug user can hire a needle and syringe or share equipment.
Skin Popping	Subcutaneous injection (injection beneath the skin).
Mainlining	Intravenous injection using the prominent vein that runs down the inside of the forearm or any others.
Chasing the Dragon	Describes the method of taking heroin by inhalation. This is usually achieved by heating the heroin powder on a piece of tinfoil and then inhaling it.
Shooting up, Jacking up, Having a fix, Fixing	Describes the ritualised aspects of the process of preparing to inject and injecting.
Cold Turkey	Describes the process of withdrawal, particularly from heroin, during which the skin may have a cold 'goose-fleshy' appearance.
Works	A term given to the equipment (needles and syringe) necessary for injecting. In a wider sense, the term may include such things as the spoon involved in heating up heroin and paraphernalia such as medical carrying cases.
Gear	This is usually used as a term covering the drug which is itself to be used for injection (usually heroin), but it may also refer to the equipment used.
Doubling up	This is the mixing of two drugs together to achieve a different effect from that obtainable from one alone.

7.2   ATTITUDES TOWARDS DRUGS AND INJECTING DRUG USE

Attitudes towards drugs vary widely between societies and at different points in history. On the whole, legal recreational drugs such as alcohol and tobacco are socially acceptable in Europe and North America today. Alcohol consumption may even be socially sanctioned by Christian religious rites. In many Islamic societies, on the other hand, alcohol is severely disapproved of. In Britain both tea and coffee have in the past been the subject of intense disapproval. In the eighteenth century, when tea-drinking first became widespread, it was attacked for having 'corrosive, gnawing and poisonous power' and for being 'a destroyer of health, an enfeebler of the frame, an engenderer of effeminacy and laziness, a debaucher of youth and a maker of misery in old age' (Cobbett, 1830). A century earlier, in a petition organised by women, coffee was accused of causing impotence and sterility, and coffee houses themselves were closed by the government for being places which encouraged sedition.

Attitudes towards so-called 'hard drugs' such as heroin and opium also vary dramatically between cultures and between different historical periods. Opiate use in Europe has been popular since the Crusades, and its uses were praised by Chaucer and Shakespeare (Whitaker, 1987). Opiates were also readily available as remedies for coughs and other minor ailments throughout nineteenth-century Britain (Berridge & Edwards, 1982). In addition, cocaine was used as a dental anaesthetic, and Conan Doyle's Sherlock Holmes found it 'transcendingly stimulating and clarifying to the mind' (Whitaker, 1987).

Why some drugs should be socially sanctioned and others disapproved of is too complex to discuss here. Suffice it to say that many substances which are harmful to the health raise substantial revenues for government via the taxes that are imposed on them. There may also be something in the claim that when drug use leads to 'undeserved' pleasures, when it gives rise to experiences that question the taken-for-granted 'reality' and when it is unrelated to productivity, it is particularly likely that social disapproval will be brought into play (Young, 1973).

Attitudes to the injection of illegal drugs contrast sharply with those towards the more legitimate kinds of injection that take place in medical contexts. Because self-injection is a specialised activity outside most people's everyday experience, negative images can be constructed around it, stereotyping those who inject as 'addicts' and 'junkies'.

7.3   A SHORT HISTORY OF INJECTING DRUG USE

When asked about the kinds of illegal drugs that can be injected, most people in Britain today are likely to think of opiates such as heroin. Opiates are, however, only one group of drugs which can be injected — amphetamines, barbiturates, cocaine and even steroids can all be taken in this way. Nevertheless, because opiates are still the primary substances injected in Britain and because the history of opiate use is well documented, it is worth considering briefly some aspects of the history of opiate injection.

Opiates

Opiates have been used since ancient times to relieve pain. Preparations of opium were originally given the name 'laudanum' and were introduced to Britain in the late seventeenth century. Opium is a sticky brown gum extracted from poppies. In 1803, a white crystalline powder was isolated from opium. It was given the name 'morphine,' derived from Morpheus the Greek god of dreams. Morphine, like all opiates, acts as a depressant on the central nervous system. In addition to relieving pain, it slows down breathing and excretion and suppresses coughing. In 1893, heroin was first produced from opium. The word 'heroin' derives from the German *heroisch* meaning 'powerful', and in addition to its value as a cough suppressant, the drug was originally believed to offer a cure for morphine addiction. Opiates are generally used in order to obliterate stress and anxiety temporarily, and to derive an immediate sensation of tranquillity, which is sometimes accompanied by delusions of invulnerability and self-empowerment.

Legislation and control

By the late nineteenth century, there was a reported 'peak of perhaps 4.59 per thousand' of the American population who were regular users of opiates (Courtwright, 1982). Legislation to control this state of affairs was introduced in 1914 with the passing of the Harrison Act (also known as the Narcotics Act). In Britain, the 1920 Dangerous Drugs Act introduced parallel controls over the import and use of opium products.

Until the early 1960s, few people in Britain were known to be dependent on opiates. In 1954, for example, only 57 such cases were known to the Home Office. In 1960, there were 94 recorded heroin users in Britain. This figure rose to 195 by 1962, and to 342 by 1964. In 1961, a government inter-departmental committee chaired by Lord Brain (known as the Brain Committee) met to review the working of the Dangerous Drugs Act. It reached the conclusion that the problem of opiate dependency was small, and that existing arrangements for control were adequate. In 1964 the Brain Committee was hastily reconvened after a further increase in the number of those dependent on opiates. Its report, published in 1965, concluded that a few physicians were responsible for 'massive inappropriate prescribing', and its recommendations led to the 1971 Misuse of Drugs Act which made new provision for the control and prosecution of drug offenders. They also led to the establishment of the Advisory Council on the Misuse of Drugs, which was given the task of keeping under review the misuse of drugs in Britain.

Until the 1970s, an arrangement known colloquially as 'the British System' operated. This used the legal prescription of drugs to identify and manage injecting drug use on the assumption that opiate dependency was an 'illness' requiring medical intervention and treatment. In the 1970s, there was a shift away from this stance towards the penal control of injecting drug use via stricter policing and the prosecution of offenders. Thereafter, injecting drug users have increasingly been viewed as criminals rather than individuals in need of care and medical attention.

A short history of hypodermic use

Drug injection predates the use of hypodermic syringes. During the seventeenth century when the injection of opium first became popular, a variety of instruments including quills and sharp wooden objects were used for the purposes of injection. Hypodermic needles did not appear until the 1840s when a Dublin doctor, Dr Rynd, described curing a patient of neuralgia by injecting him with acetate of morphine. The hypodermic treatment of battle injuries during the American Civil War (1861–1865) was a catalyst which led to widespread use.

The term 'hypodermic' (originally 'ipodermic') originated from the work of Dr Charles Hunter who in 1867 was one of the first to investigate the 'general therapeutic effect' that followed from the injection of morphine. This early research contributed to an uncritical acceptance of the marvellous benefits of hypodermic administration. A commentator at the time proclaimed excitedly, 'Of danger there is absolutely none ... the advantages of hypodermic injection of morphine over its administration by mouth are immense.'

7.4 INJECTING DRUG USE IN BRITAIN TODAY

Accurate statistics concerning the number of injecting drug users in Britain today are hard to come by. In 1988, Home Office estimates put the number of people regularly injecting heroin in the region of 50,000, with about 10,000 people injecting other drugs. These figures may, of course, be underestimates because they are calculated on the basis of those who are known to official agencies, those who are registered for therapy and those who are known to the police. Calculating the number of users becomes even more complicated if a distinction is made between people who inject regularly and those who do so recreationally or occasionally. Estimates suggest that about the same number of individuals may inject occasionally as do so regularly (Robertson, 1987).

Injection tends to be an urban phenomenon (Pearson, 1987b). In Glasgow, for example, it is estimated that '8,000 to 12,000 – mainly among the unemployed on the peripheral housing estates' currently inject (Steed, 1987). Estimates of the prevalence of injecting drug use change rapidly, and there may also be significant local variations on the national pattern. In Edinburgh, it has recently been reported that the wave of heroin use which swept the city's housing estates in 1983 appears to be receding, with local doctors estimating that heroin use has dropped by a third (Steed, 1987).

The drugs which users take, the means by which they are taken, the frequency and the amount that is injected vary greatly from one area to another. In Edinburgh, for example, heroin injection has been reported as being particularly prevalent, whereas in Liverpool smoking heroin has been reported as more common. These variations may relate to the relative purity of the drug used as well as its availability.

In some situations, heroin may not be the primary drug injected, with amphetamines and cocaine being injected in preference to it. Some injectors may prefer to inject a combination of amphetamines and opiates, and others may switch between drugs if their chosen drug is unavailable. In some areas, steroids may also be injected, perhaps in connection with involvement in sports such as weight training. These users may be involved in a completely different 'drug culture' to other injectors. It is important to recognise that, regardless of the drug injected, the risk of HIV transmission if needles and syringes are shared is just as great.

Unhelpful stereotypes hinder an accurate understanding of injecting drug use in Britain today. These tend to suggest that all injecting drug users are young, working class and unemployed. In reality, those who inject drugs are as varied as the rest of the population, there being no such thing as a 'typical drug user'. Heroin and other illegal drugs may be injected in affluent penthouses or run-down inner city estates. Popular stereotypes of injecting drug use may be further influenced by the relative invisibility of certain kinds of users. Older and more well-to-do injectors, for example, may obtain their supplies and equipment through channels which enable them to escape surveillance by the police and drugs agencies.

7.5   GENDER, SEXUALITY AND INJECTING DRUG USE

Gender and sexuality need to be considered for a number of reasons when thinking about injecting drug use and HIV infection. Some of these relate to the fact that HIV can be transmitted sexually between those who inject. Others concern the specific problems that may confront women who inject, and women and men who involve themselves in prostitution as a way of paying for their supplies.

A series of specific problems confront women injectors (DAWN, 1985). These vary from the different way in which society evaluates injecting drug use amongst women and men to the particular difficulties women may face in using drug dependency facilities. On the whole, society views women who inject drugs more negatively than men. They are frequently perceived as 'mad' or 'sick' rather than as people who have simply broken the law. Beliefs such as these often inform decisions about the custody of children. It is by no means uncommon for a woman who injects to lose the custody of her children once her status as a drug user has become known (Stewart, 1987). Similar issues can arise in connection with pregnancy, when pressure may be put (either implicity or explicity) on the woman concerned to have an abortion irrespective of her own wishes. Other problems may arise if a woman decides against a termination and if she is concurrently receiving methadone as part of a substitution or maintenance programme (see Section 7.7). While prescribed drugs may have an advantage in terms of purity over street heroin, women's organisations have pointed out that heroin may be less dangerous to the foetus than methadone (DAWN, 1987).

A rather different set of issues can arise in connection with women's use of drug dependency facilities. These frequently have a male-dominated atmosphere – in some cases, over 80% of clients may be men – which can be oppressive and alienating for many women. Since few drugs agencies cater specifically for women's needs, women drug users often have to rely on their own alternative support networks to cope with problems linked to drug use. Family and friends as well as other women drug users may be more commonly relied upon than is the case with male drug users.

Some women may turn to prostitution as a means of paying for drugs, and male partners may encourage this as a means of paying for their own supplies. For other women, prostitution may offer a means of maintaining their drug use in a way which is more controllable than criminal activity, although prostitutes continuously face the risk of arrest for soliciting. Whilst many prostitutes prefer only to have safer sex, their risk of acquiring HIV infection may be increased because some clients offer higher payment for sex without a condom.

Male injecting drug users involved in prostitution are almost invariably portrayed as gay, but it is important to realise that many of those who participate in homosexual acts may retain a heterosexual identity. Contrary to popular belief, prostitution is not restricted to men who identify themselves as gay, nor to women who identify themselves as heterosexual.

Lesbians who inject drugs may be further cut off from mainstream provision by drug welfare schemes. They tend to face many of the same problems as other women who are injecting drug users but may encounter additional difficulties stemming from general insensitivity and hostility towards lesbianism.

7.6   HOMELESSNESS

For many injecting drug users, particularly those who are young, homelessness can be a problem. Drug agencies report that it is often difficult to find accommodation for drug users, as landlords and other residents may show prejudice. The problem of homelessness for young lesbians and young gay men can be acute since they may have been rejected by their families and, as both drug users and as either lesbian or gay, they may face additional prejudice.

7.7 CONVENTIONAL INTERVENTIONS

A number of different approaches to the regulation of injecting drug use have been attempted. In recent years, two different systems of intervention have co-existed somewhat uneasily alongside each other. The first of these, the 'British System', aims to regulate drug use by providing a legal supply of substitute drugs to replace reliance on illegal sources. The ultimate goal of this approach is usually either detoxification or maintenance. A second strategy, which until recently has been more widely used in the United States, aims to control drug use by tougher police action and penal sanction. An excellent discussion of these two systems can be found in a recent article by Malyon (1986).

Throughout the 1960s and 1970s, drugs policy in Britain was influenced by the view that injecting drug use could be regulated via substitution, detoxification and maintenance, and a number of different forms of provision emerged in response to this (MacGregor & Ettorre, 1987). These include Drug Dependency Units (DDUs), Street Agencies and Rehabilitation Units.

DDU provision varies across the country, although most are linked to major hospitals. In some areas, very few DDUs exist, whereas in others there may be many units. Nearly all DDUs operate on a catchment area basis, and most have a waiting list. Many require patients to be referred to them by a GP. The treatment provided by DDUs varies considerably. Some only offer out-patient treatment, others only offer in-patient detoxification, and several will not prescribe drugs. Doctors working in DDUs are obliged to notify the Home Office of those they treat.

Some terms explained

Substitution

Under the 'British System', Methadone (a drug which to some extent mimics the effects of heroin) was introduced as a form of *substitution* therapy. Methadone has a similar effect to heroin, although it has less of a tendency to produce euphoria. It can be taken either orally, or in the form of injectable physeptone, and has a longer effect than heroin. Methadone dependency is built up more slowly, but lasts longer.

Maintenance

Methadone can also be prescribed in a long-term programme of *maintenance*. The aim here is to offer the user a safer form of drug use for an unspecified period, perhaps until any underlying problems have been resolved. While positive results were initially ascribed to Methadone maintenance therapy, long-term evaluation has suggested that it has few

---

if any 'curative' effects. Methadone withdrawal is felt by some users to be more difficult physically than heroin withdrawal. This may be because of the drug's synthetic nature and the slower rate at which it is broken down in the body.

Detoxification

Detoxification operates from the assumption that physical withdrawal is the hardest aspect to deal with in giving up heroin use. In a detoxification programme, Methadone is often prescribed on a reducing basis for a short period (up to 12 weeks) to assist in an initial process of *detoxification*. Following this, the drug is withdrawn completely.

The second group of organisations are the Street Agencies. These tend to be at least partly funded by health authorities and local authorities and are community-based in their operation. They offer counselling, information and advice, and a community nurse and social worker are usually attached. Where there is a doctor involved, she or he is obliged to notify the Home Office about those attending for treatment, but the other workers are not. Some Street Agencies offer medication as part of their service; others do not but instead seek to arrange GP support for their clients. Most can refer clients on for in-patient treatment. Workers will usually accept immediate self-referral and make home visits.

The third kind of drugs organisation is the Rehabilitation Unit. Clients usually have to be drug-free before they can be offered help by this kind of facility whose aim is to reintegrate drug users into mainstream society. Rehabilitation Units are usually residential but may be run in very different ways. Some, for example, take the form of therapeutic communities. These often have a hierarchical structure which residents have to work their way up as time passes. A number of therapeutic communities have a commitment to intensive confrontational group sessions during which members of the community will encourage and berate one another. Other rehabilitation units may be founded on a religious conviction. Organisationally, these latter units vary, with religion being more central to the concept of therapy in some of them than in others. Finally, there are Generalist Rehabilitation Units which operate on more democratic principles. Group and individual support may be provided in these, and residents may be encouraged to take a positive role in determining the nature of their therapy.

The 1970s and 1980s, however, have seen increased demands for a 'toughening up' of principles and procedures in line with the view that injecting drug use can be controlled through more aggressive policing and heavier fines for the sale and possession of drugs. Following this change of emphasis, the number of drug users receiving custodial sentences rose by 21% in 1984 to reach nearly 5,000. Recently, there have also been retrospective prosecutions for the possession of illegal drugs. This kind of intervention led to the trial of the singer Boy George in 1986 for the past possession of heroin. Whether this style of intervention will be more successful than other strategies in restricting the use of illegal drugs remains to be seen.

7.8   NEW INITIATIVES

As has been explained earlier, the sharing of needles and syringes can be a major means of HIV transmission, as can be sexual intercourse with an infected person who injects. HIV is not, however, the only infection that can be transmitted via blood-to-blood contact — other diseases such as hepatitis B have long been known to be transmitted in this way. Candida albicans infection (thrush), transmitted through shared syringes, is also widespread in certain areas, causing eye infections such as endophthalmitis (Robertson, 1987), and between 1982 and 1984, unexplained outbreaks of heart valve disease occurred amongst injecting drug users in New York and in Britain. These episodes subsequently faded and no full explanation of their cause has been given, although a blood-borne infectious agent transmitted via shared needles and syringes has been suspected.

Since HIV infection has become a significant health threat among injecting drug users, health educators have been prompted to consider the most appropriate interventions to restrict the further spread of infection. Some new initiatives emphasise *harm minimisation*. By aiming to reduce the risks associated with unsafe injecting techniques, a number of interventions of this kind have offered advice on how best to clean needles and syringes between use. Others have taken a more radical stance by supplying injecting drug users with supplies of clean needles and syringes. Both of these kinds of intervention increasingly recognise the need to combine information about safer injecting technique with guidance about safer sex.

Syringe and needle exchange schemes

In December 1986, following a review of options for preventing the further spread of HIV infection among injecting drug users, drug agencies were granted £1 million to enhance their counselling services and to establish a number of syringe and needle exchange schemes. Fifteen agencies in England and Scotland were initially recruited to take part in an assessment of the usefulness of this kind of harm minimisation strategy.

These centres distribute needles and syringes, sometimes on an exchange basis, and sometimes on request. Depending on the needs of the individual as well as on the policy of the particular centre, anything from one needle and one syringe up to forty needles and syringes may be made available on one occasion, often with a 'sharps' container or box to be used for storing used equipment before it is returned to the exchange. A number of centres also distribute other equipment to satisfy drug users' needs: for example, ampoules of sterile water and alcohol pads to help drug users improve their injecting technique, and different sized syringes and needles. In addition to making sterile equipment available, some syringe and needle exchange schemes offer advice on the steps that can be taken as a last resort to clean equipment between use. They may also provide counselling about safer sex and condom use.

Secondary health issues such as the prevention of infection and other health problems connected with poor injection technique have also been tackled by some exchange schemes. In a number of centres, advice is given on better injection technique. This may help users identify the most accessible parts of the body as well as the importance of using multiple sites. Poor injection technique has often presented users with general health problems including abscesses, phlebitis, bruising and thrombosed veins. Advice may also be given on the most appropriate ways of preparing a drug for injection. This can include counselling users about the importance of using clean water when preparing drugs for use.

Criticisms

There have of course been many criticisms of the implementation of harm-reduction strategies such as these. When syringe exchange schemes were first considered, doubts were expressed about their legality. In Scotland, for example, it was originally feared that those working in them might find themselves subject to criminal prosecution for the common law offence of reckless conduct, and it was not until the Lord Advocate let it be known that as long as staff followed accepted procedures they would remain immune from prosecution, that this matter was resolved.

It is still the case, however, that clients using exchange schemes may be liable to prosecution if traces of an illegal substance are found within the hypodermic syringes they return for exchange, but the Attorney General has recently announced that, 'when reaching decisions in cases relating to the misuse of drugs, the Crown Prosecution Service, where relevant, will have proper regard to public interest considerations arising out of the measures being brought in to halt the spread of the AIDS virus' (Hansard, 1987). A number of centres report that the police are using increased discretion in monitoring their activity and, in some places, people found with used syringes from an exchange scheme are issued with a receipt if their equipment is confiscated, to enable them to claim fresh supplies.

Criticisms of exchange schemes have also come from those who suggest that most young people have neither tried nor plan to try illegal drugs. Giving information and providing free syringes, it is argued, may stimulate a demand for injectable drugs and actually promote the problem it seeks to solve. In areas of the country where the injection of drugs is infrequent in comparison to drug taking by other means, some people have argued that there is no need for syringe exchange programmes. To introduce them in these circumstances could be to alter the situation in a particular locality and therefore to increase the risks of HIV transmission.

Syringe and needle exchange — a success?

Evidence in support of harm minimisation as a viable way of reducing the incidence of HIV infection comes from statistics showing high levels of HIV seropositivity amongst injecting drug users in areas where syringe availability has traditionally been strictly controlled. In Edinburgh, for example, prior to the introduction of a syringe exchange scheme, the police had campaigned to get chemists not to sell syringes to suspected illegal injecting drug users. By way of contrast, during 1984, an estimated 13,000 syringes were reported to have been distributed by chemists in London (Robertson, 1987). HIV infection rates amongst injecting drug users have been reported as significantly higher in Edinburgh than in London. Similar findings emerge from studies comparing the situation in New York where syringe availability has been severely restricted, with that in Amsterdam where there have been long-running syringe exchange programmes (Robertson, 1987).

Although chemists in some parts of Britain have been pressured not to sell syringes, in most places they can still be bought over the counter. Syringe exchange schemes, on the other hand, have the advantage of being able to provide drug users with advice and support as well as free syringes. For society, a positive aspect of syringe exchange programmes is that syringes are usually returned and disposed of without risk to anyone else. There is no guarantee that this will occur with syringes bought from chemists.

There are a number of evaluation studies of exchange schemes currently underway, although at the moment only their preliminary findings are available (Stimson, 1989).

7.9   CONCLUSIONS

It is essential for health educators to understand drug use because unsafe injecting practices can be a major route of HIV transmission. In order to deal with unhelpful stereotypes and prejudice about injecting drug use, it is also important to appreciate wider social attitudes towards drug use. In particular, it is unhelpful to assume within the context of AIDS education that injecting drug users are in some way too weak to cope with their own problems. An awareness is also needed of broader social factors such as gender, sexuality, unemployment and homelessness, which may themselves be exacerbated by both personal and institutionalised prejudice towards injecting drug use. It should also be recognised that injecting drug use may be just one indication of a wider-ranging set of personal and social problems confronting the individual.

Finally, it is important for health educators to realise that just as 'safer sex' can reduce the risk of HIV transmission through sexual activity, 'safer drug-related practices' can do the same with respect to HIV transmission through injection. By following harm-reduction guidelines, and by taking care not to share their equipment with other people, injecting drug users can dramatically reduce the risk of HIV infection through their injecting practices.

References

Berridge, V. & Edwards, G. (1982) *Opium and the People – opiate use in 19th-century England* New York, St Martin's Press.

Cobbett, W. (1830) *Rural Rides* (1967 ed), Harmondsworth, Penguin Books.

Courtwright, D.T. (1982) *Dark Paradise: opiate addiction in America before 1940*, Cambridge, Mass., Harvard University Press.

DAWN (1985) *A Survey of Facilities for Women Using Drugs (including Alcohol) in London*, London, Drugs Alcohol Women Nationally.

DAWN (1987) *Women and Heroin and other Opiates*, London, Drugs Alcohol Women Nationally.

Hansard (1987), Cited in *Druglink*, May–June 1987, London ISDD.

ISDD (1987) Heroin today: commodity, consumption, control and care, in N. Dorn & N. South (eds) *A Land Fit for Heroin?* London, Macmillan.

McGachy, C. (1985) *Deviant Behaviour: crime, conflict and interest groups*, New York, Macmillan.

MacGregor, S. & Ettoree, B. (1987) From treatment to rehabilitation – aspects of the evolution of British policy on the care of drug-takers, in N. Dorn & N. South (eds) *A Land Fit for Heroin?* London, Macmillan.

Malyon, T. (1986) Full tilt towards a no-win 'Vietnam' war on drugs, *New Statesman*, 17 October. pp 7–10.

Pearson, G. (1987a) *The New Heroin Users*, Oxford, Blackwell.

Pearson, G. (1987b) Social deprivation, unemployment and patterns of heroin use, in N. Dorn & N. South (eds) *A Land Fit for Heroin?* London, Macmillan.

Robertson, R. (1987) *Heroin, AIDS and Society*, London, Hodder & Stoughton.

Steed, J. (1987) Article in *Guardian*, 3 January.

Stewart, T. (1987) *The Heroin Users*, London, Pandora Press.

Stimson, G. (1989) Syringe exchange schemes in England and Scotland, in P. Aggleton, G. Hart & P. Davies (eds) *AIDS: Social Representations and Social Practices*, Lewes, Falmer Press.

Whitaker, B. (1987) *The Global Connection*, London, Jonathan Cape.

Young, J. (1973) The amplification of drug use, in S. Cohen & J. Young (eds) *The Manufacture of News: deviance, social problems and the mass media*, London, Constable.

8.   Living with HIV infection, living with AIDS

Earlier chapters in this book have been concerned with medical, scientific and social issues. It is important, however, to remember the personal dimension and that, as with any other condition, 'the disease and the patient are not the same thing' (Malcolmson, 1988). Whilst health education about AIDS is obviously needed to explain the nature, modes of transmission and natural history of HIV infection, it must also be able to communicate the experience of those who are diagnosed with HIV infection and its various consequences.

A wide range of psychological and social considerations will affect an individual's experience of HIV or AIDS. These vary from the individual's previous attitudes towards health issues to the availability or otherwise of adequate local health-care provision. Moreover, the way in which someone was initially infected may have much bearing on subsequent events. In this respect, the experience of haemophiliacs may be very different from that of injecting drug users or gay men. Geographical factors may also be important. The proximity of the individual to local voluntary sector support groups may affect how they cope with HIV infection or AIDS.

Nevertheless, everyone with HIV infection is likely to be equally affected by the cultural associations that still prevail in Britain. Infected people not only face an uncertain future, but also widespread ignorance, fear and prejudice. Most people who are ill take it for granted that they can discuss their condition with their family and friends, but people with HIV infection may feel unable to discuss their situation even with those who were previously closest to them, for fear of being rejected or discriminated against. They may be condemned to silence on the very subject which they most need to talk about, at a time when they feel most afraid and insecure.

Emphasis on the mortality rates of people with AIDS has produced an atmosphere of unparalleled fatalism concerning the syndrome. Widespread victim-blaming has also added to the difficulties encountered by many people with HIV infection or AIDS. These same factors can also affect the families, lovers, friends and health-care providers who live with or support them. As one commentator has observed, in this context intellectual sophistication is no antidote to fear (Cooke, 1987). Moreover, while society is beginning to learn to live with HIV infection and its consequences, an understanding of the epidemic has not been helped by a continued tendency in the media to sensationalise and offer conflicting messages about the ways in which the virus is and is not transmitted. Health educators should therefore recognise that for some time to come they will be working with large numbers of the 'worried well': people whose anxieties, though largely unfounded, may be only too real. They should therefore aim to dispel the morbid fatalism that surrounds and informs both lay and professional perceptions of HIV infection and AIDS.

8.1 LIVING WITH HIV

Fortunately, many people who discover they are HIV antibody positive will have received counselling before and after their test result. Nevertheless, people who have recently been diagnosed are likely to experience a wide range of emotional responses, from shock and anger, to frustration and feelings of guilt. Although they may not necessarily feel 'unwell', people with HIV infection are likely to live with considerable uncertainty. For those with PGL, there may be the ever-present reminder of swollen lymph nodes, and for everyone there is the possibility that the signs and symptoms that others take for granted as evidence of a cough or cold may, for them, be the first evidence of more serious, and possibly life-threatening disease.

It is therefore important for people with HIV infection to be offered the opportunity to join and participate in the numerous support groups that are growing up around Britain. The sometimes overwhelming sense of uncertainty that can accompany the initial diagnosis requires and deserves experienced counselling. Within the context of Body Positive groups (see Appendix C) or other equivalent organisations, this can often be provided by people who have the infection itself but have learned how to accept and live with their diagnosis.

Health educators will need to explore with others the ways in which the needs of people with HIV infection may differ depending on how they came to be infected. For example, transfusion recipients who find themselves infected as a direct consequence of medical treatment may feel 'a sense of betrayal and a lack of trust both in the medical establishment and in themselves for having made a choice to take a particular course of treatment. In such a situation, the ability to attribute blame to an outside source, such as the medical establishment, can be a very useful coping tool for the individual and should not be taken from them' (Deitch, 1987). As a result, 'helping professionals must be prepared to hear and understand what may sometimes be some disturbing degrees of anger towards them' (Deitch, 1987). Moreover, unlike others with HIV infection, 'transfusion recipients are unique in so far as they do not maintain as part of their identity the fact that they *were* transfusion recipients' (Deitch, 1987).

The situation of transfusion recipients may be very different from that of injecting drug users and gay men who may blame themselves for having become infected. Resolving these feelings of self-recrimination may often be the first step towards a renewed self-confidence and sense of self-esteem.

Health educators should also be sensitive to the stress that can follow a positive HIV test result and recognise that responses to stress vary considerably, as do the strategies individuals use to cope with it. Consequently, people with HIV infection need and deserve a great deal of individualised support in order to help them come to terms with their position. Exercise, good diet, friendship and the opportunity to share deep and conflicting emotions are all important factors in learning to live with HIV.

Women may experience HIV infection very differently from men: 'Most seropositive women experience social isolation. For some, this isolation comes from a lack of a specifically defined community with which to identify. For others, the mistaken belief that AIDS organisations provide services only to gay men prevents them from seeking help' (Blachman, 1988). Women with HIV infection can gain considerable emotional support by meeting others in a similar position, and from sharing the pain and sadness which may perhaps come from the fear of transmitting the virus to their children, the fear of leaving their children motherless and the fear of pregnancy with its possible consequences. Counselling may support women through these difficulties and help them to make choices about their futures.

A negative HIV antibody test result can also have long-term social and emotional consequences, due to the individual having recognised that AIDS is indeed a concrete reality and a possible threat to health. Individual responses to a negative test result may be complicated by the fact that a friend or lover has already tested positive. The question 'Why them but not me?' can cause stress, especially in relationships where one partner is HIV antibody negative and the other HIV antibody positive. Some seronegative people may experience a degree of 'survivor guilt', particularly if they have friends and acquaintances who are seropositive. Occasionally, a negative test result can lead people to withdraw from everyday social life and from sexual relationships, perhaps through fear of HIV infection. Reactions like these can be exaggerated by the anxiety which inevitably accompanies the delay between taking the test and receiving the result. It is important therefore to provide opportunities for HIV seronegative people to discuss their feelings and, if necessary, seek expert advice. People who become HIV seropositive after a previously negative test result often find it particularly difficult to come to terms with their changed antibody status and are likely to need sustained support and counselling.

8.2 LIVING WITH ARC

Being diagnosed with ARC is likely to be a very distressing experience, especially for those who have just learned to live with asymptomatic HIV infection. ARC refers to a wide variety of conditions, ranging from herpes zoster (shingles) to night sweats or persistent diarrhoea. Long-term fatigue and weight-loss may also impair a person's ability to cope with her or his diagnosis of ARC. People with ARC are understandably worried that they may develop AIDS. This uncertainty is often more difficult to handle than the actual symptoms, even when the latter are severe. Because of this, people with ARC sometimes have a strong resistance to participating in groups offering support to people with AIDS. They may thus become socially isolated.

The experience of individuals with ARC differs considerably depending on the degree and duration of episodes of ill-health. Nevertheless, in all cases, it is important for health professionals and others to be sensitive to practical problems concerning housing, finance, employment and access to social services that many people with ARC face.

As with all forms of periodic illness, many people in this position may benefit from efforts to help them maintain their everyday lives with dignity. There is an advocacy role here for health-care professionals to support people with ARC in their efforts to resist discrimination and prejudice.

8.3   LIVING WITH AIDS

Whilst many can cope intellectually with the idea that AIDS is a syndrome made up of many distinct conditions, it is perhaps harder to accept that AIDS can be experienced in many different ways. The sequence and combination of the wide range of opportunistic diseases that make up the syndrome means that individual people with AIDS may share little or no direct experience of symptoms or treatments with one another. The situation of a person with Kaposi's sarcoma may thus be very different from that of someone recovering from Pneumocystis carinii pneumonia. The experience of someone diagnosed with AIDS 'out of the blue' may be very different from that of another person who previously knew they were HIV seropositive, or had PGL or ARC.

Many people with AIDS also face the difficult task of informing family and friends of their diagnosis at the same time as they break the news that they are an injecting drug user, or gay, or possibly both. One man with AIDS has described how he initially decided *not* to tell his family: 'For me the issues were simple. The unselfish one was that I didn't want to hurt them. The selfish (and more valid) one was that I knew my parents well. They'd get totally hysterical, if not physically ill, and make it "their" problem, forcing me to take care of them when I was the one who had the problem and needed to be taken care of most. I decided that if and when I became really sick, they'd have to know, and that would be soon enough.' However, he did in the end tell his parents, since in the event he was 'overwhelmed by the very stress I was trying to avoid by not telling them' (Russo, 1988). Paradoxically, many people with AIDS have described how they have ended up caring for those close to them who find the diagnosis hard to accept. Whilst this may place a seemingly unfair burden on some, others have found it a positive means of dealing with their own situation, recognising that they still exercise power and responsibility in their lives as people with AIDS.

The British organisation Frontliners offers the following advice to the recently diagnosed facing this dilemma: 'If you feel comfortable with the idea and your parents are likely to be supportive, then you should tell them you have AIDS. On the other hand, if you feel the news might alienate them or if you feel they might find the situation too stressful, then perhaps you should consider not telling them for the time being. Don't rush into any course of action until you have thought through the consequences. You are the best judge of what to do. You know your family better than anyone else' (Frontliners, 1987). Individuals facing this situation are invited to ask themselves the following questions:

– Will it be even more of a worry to you if you do not tell your parents?
– If you should die without having told your family, how would they feel?
– Might they feel even more hurt because they would have wanted to help?
– Might they react against your lover and friends who did know?

[Frontliners, 1987]

As health education challenges myths and stereotypes about AIDS, the situation of people with AIDS will doubtless improve. In the meantime, although their medical and clinical status may differ, people with AIDS still experience the consequences of the widespread ignorance, hostility and prejudice surrounding their condition. Organising to support one another and to provide counselling and other services for friends and families, many people with AIDS have developed a strong social identity, based on their collective determination to affirm the dignity and value of their lives, together with a desire to resist attacks on civil liberties.

Many people are surprised to learn that people with AIDS spend most of their time living in the community. As Jones (1986) has pointed out, 'Although many of the opportunistic infections that occur as a result of the compromised immunity of AIDS need energetic in-patient therapy, most symptoms are dealt with at home.' Contrary to popular belief, people with AIDS are rarely bed-ridden for long periods of time — the syndrome is characterised by periods of severe illness interspersed by periods of relative remission. Nevertheless, everyone with AIDS lives with the constant stress of knowing that they may become seriously ill at any time. They also face the possibility of HIV encephalopathy and its psychological consequences. Whilst it is important to recognise that people with AIDS are not merely passive and powerless 'victims' or 'sufferers', AIDS is frequently an extremely harrowing and physically painful disease. Drug treatments too may have unpleasant and debilitating side effects which may add to the stress associated with the syndrome.

It is therefore important for people with AIDS to be encouraged to accept and acknowledge their medical diagnosis. At the same time, this 'acceptance' and 'acknowledgement' can have many faces. As one person with AIDS has written, 'hopelessness can exist side by side with love and compassion. We may be better people if we can allow these ideas room to flourish' (Zachar, 1987). It is certainly not helpful for health-care providers to pretend that AIDS is anything other than a frequently terrible and, as yet, incurable condition.

Nevertheless, people with AIDS can be helped to make informed choices concerning most aspects of their everyday lives. These include making provision for their eventual death and making decisions about life-sustaining treatments which may take place after the person concerned is mentally unable to participate in decision-making. Above all, people with AIDS need trust in themselves and in others around them. As one such person has put it, 'I would say that the most important thing to hold on to is a belief in yourself, the ability to make your own decisions. You can't put all your trust in professionals. I mean, unless you find a doctor who's willing to work with you, explain things to you and give you options. Knowledge is power, which means you have to remain very sceptical of things people tell you. It means you have to get a broad range of views, different opinions' (Berkowitz, 1986).

It may also be salutary for health educators to reflect on the view that 'one aspect of professionals, whether it's health care or mental care or whatever, is that too many of them believe that they have to always appear to have the answers — that they have to seem cool and in control. The best hope that you can have is to talk to people, to remain sceptical, to educate yourself as much as you can and to get maybe as many opinions as you can and to really, you know, take your time before you make any decisions whatsoever' (Berkowitz, 1986). In such ways, AIDS may become less associated with death, and more concerned with a positive and affirmative identity.

Sadly, a number of health-care professionals seem out of touch with specialist thinking on AIDS, and in a recent survey of GPs, only 16% surveyed showed a 'good' or 'very good' knowledge of the syndrome (Boyton & Scambler, 1988). Moreover, given the time delay between infection and the appearance of symptoms, it is likely to be some time before most GPs have direct experience of AIDS in the course of their everyday work. Health education will therefore be particulary important for those on the 'frontline' of care — home helps, psychiatric social workers, voluntary sector 'buddies' and community-based health networks. This is especially important in relation to families with children with AIDS, where both the child and the rest of the family may need extensive help and support. Since about 20% of people with AIDS can now expect to live for two years or more after the initial diagnosis, it is important for health educators to examine the processes by which AIDS comes to be commonly understood as an immediately fatal condition. Health-care providers will also need to be aware of the different ways in which individuals assimilate their diagnosis into their everyday lives, especially when physical disfigurement may be involved. In this situation, 'the distinction between pain and suffering is an important point to emphasise. Pain does not mean suffering, nor does suffering come from pain alone' (Schofferman, 1987).

8.4 AIDS IN THE COMMUNITY: PLANNING FOR THE FUTURE

The epidemiology of HIV infection and AIDS in Britain identifies the specific groups most directly affected by the epidemic (see Sections 2.3 and 2.4). With present estimates suggesting that between 40,000 and 100,000 people in Britain may be infected, future levels of demand on public services are likely to be enormous. The management of HIV infection and AIDS also raises complex issues to do with housing, welfare provision and community support. A district medical officer involved in planning has recently stated that 'the biggest hurdle we have to overcome is in relation to public moral attitudes towards the largest risk group, homosexuals. The "wrath of God" and "divine retribution" views have been over-publicised, and there are undoubtedly many people, our NHS staff among them, who share these attitudes' (Crown, 1987). In consequence, 'a prime task therefore for service providers at present is the development of sensitive and balanced education programmes, which address not only the information needs of staff and carers, but also their attitudes.' Fortunately, health education officers with a special responsibility for education about HIV infection and AIDS have been appointed by many health authorities and local authorities throughout Britain. Their work is vital if people with AIDS are to receive the same standards of care and welfare provision as others who are ill.

Welfare benefits

The welfare benefits available to people with HIV infection and/or AIDS depend like everybody else's on the individual's previous history of employment, National Insurance contributions, and the length and extent of illness. If an employer does not provide sick pay, sickness benefit may be available from the Department of Social Security, depending on National Insurance contributions. Other forms of benefit are also available, including Invalidity Pensions, and Severe Disablement Allowances (SDA), Disablement Benefits, Mobility and Attendance Allowances, Supplementary Benefits, and special diet and heating allowances. Up-to-date information on these allowances can be obtained from the Terrence Higgins Trust and other voluntary sector organisations.

Employment

Unlike the United States and some European countries, Britain has not passed laws to prevent discrimination against people with HIV infection or AIDS. Sadly, irrational fears have been widely amplified by the media, and until public understanding of the virus's specific and very limited modes of transmission improves, it seems likely that prejudice will remain. Current employment legislation gives someone who has been employed for two years or more (one year for those who started work before 1 June 1985 in firms which employ more than twenty people) the right to apply to an industrial tribunal if they feel they have been dismissed unfairly. The Department of Employment (DE) has concluded that 'Dismissing individuals who are infected, or thought to be infected, simply because of pressure from other employees would in many cases expose the employer to a claim for unfair dismissal' (DE, 1987). In order to prevent situations like these arising, the DE recommends participatory health education in the workplace.

Housing

The advent of AIDS has highlighted once again the inability of all sectors of housing to meet the needs of people with serious health problems (RIS, 1987). Loss of income, discrimination or physical disability can lead some people with HIV infection and its consequences to become homeless at a time when stability and security are especially important. Home owners with mortgages may find it difficult to keep up their repayments and should inform their bank and building society before the problem gets out of hand. It may be possible to renegotiate the terms on which repayments are made. The Department of Social Security may also offer assistance with the payment of interest on mortgages if the individual concerned is unemployed and in receipt of income support, but they will not repay any part of the capital. In appropriate circumstances, claims can also be made for help with the payment of water rates, ground rent, essential maintenance and insurance.

In the unfortunate event of homelessness, local authorities have a statutory obligation under Section 3 of the 1985 Housing Act to give priority to applicants for housing if they are vulnerable due to ill health or disability. Harassment, domestic violence and the physical inadequacy of accommodation can also be grounds for application to local authority housing departments. In such circumstances, 'confidentiality policies should always be maintained. There is no reason why information concerning HIV status should be passed on to anyone else, including other staff in the authority, even if they may be directly involved with the applicant. Speed in providing assistance is of the essence and a medical assessment should be made as quickly as possible. Prolonged stress or living in unsatisfactory conditions can only exacerbate the problem. Above all, flexibility is required in assessing the needs and providing assistance which positively helps the applicant' (RIS, 1987).

Housing associations and voluntary organisations have an important contribution to make in the establishment of self-contained housing projects to meet the special needs of people with ARC and AIDS, and in the years ahead, local authorities cannot rely on the private sector to resolve the difficult problems that will arise in connection with homelessness and disability among those affected. Certainly, the needs of the terminally ill and the dying cannot be met by the capacity of current and projected AIDS hospice accommodation.

Community care

Tony Newton, as Minister of Health, has recently pointed out that 'whatever our success in educating people how to avoid infection with HIV, sadly we shall see thousands more cases of AIDS among those who are already infected. These will be mostly young people, who will need care and support in the face of an often debilitating, and ultimately fatal condition' (Newton, 1987). He made it clear that 'the development of a network of services and support for people with AIDS is a challenge for voluntary agencies, for the National Health

Service and for local authorities,' adding that, 'there is a consensus that services should, as far as possible, be provided to enable people to be cared for in their own homes. The task now is to develop appropriate services on the ground.'

Hospital outpatient care for people with AIDS is still in the early stages of development, but will increasingly function as a bridge between hospital services and community care (Williams, 1987). Local authorities already co-ordinate the work of health services, social services and voluntary organisations in many parts of London. Local authorities will also have to develop clear policies concerning people with AIDS, including making provision for children with AIDS and the children of people who die from AIDS (Platt, 1987). The need for long-term funding for local-government AIDS initiatives is therefore a priority. It is also important for local authorities to liaise fully with different racial and ethnic communities, and to confront racism and homophobia as and when they arise, especially in relation to welfare provision.

Given that most people with AIDS will spend perhaps 80% of the time between diagnosis and death in the community, it is clear that the training and appointment of community-based primary health-care teams should be a national priority (HMSO, 1987). As a London-based health liaison officer has recently put it, 'Preparedness, consistency and client-centredness are some of the key principles for developing local strategies. [AIDS] is a public health issue, not a moral issue. It will require resources, imagination, goodwill and determination. It is not going to go away' (Rayner, 1987).

The membership of these teams should include doctors, health visitors, district nurses, social workers, community psychiatric nurses and others. In addition to managing the community care of people with AIDS, teams like these can also support carers at home - be they families, friends or volunteers. Caring for people with AIDS is often hard work, both physically and emotionally, and it is therefore important for carers to be aware of the individuals and agencies who can support them in their work (Anon. 1987). These range from continence advisers, opticians, interpreters, physio-therapists to care attendants, sitting and minding services, meals on wheels and home adaptation services. It is within these networks of community support that the quality of life for people with AIDS can be sustained (Kohner, 1988).

It is also important for people with HIV infection and/or AIDS, their friends, lovers and families to be in contact with local voluntary sector AIDS organisations. There are already more than eighty of these in Britain, and the range of services they provide can in many cases complement that offered by statutory agencies.

8.5 DEATH AND BEREAVEMENT

Cannadine (1981), a historian who has looked at modern attitudes to death, has observed that 'death as analysed in the second half of the twentieth century is either general or in the future, or individual and in the present. It is rarely, if ever, both together.' AIDS has inexorably altered this judgement. Whilst we should beware of a tendency to idealise a mythical and non-existent past in which it might be supposed that these matters were coped with more efficiently than they are today, we should recognise that nothing has prepared us for the reality of AIDS.

In the months and years ahead, health-care providers and others must learn to be cheerful but realistic in their work with people with AIDS. Physical contact is extremely important, together with general loving care. This can become difficult as AIDS progresses, and patients become demanding and perhaps hostile. Some of these personality changes may be part of the disease. As one doctor has written:

'Care of people with AIDS is difficult. There is far too little that we can do in the face of what often seems a relentless destruction of mind and body. Despite the difficulties of the work, many doctors, nurses, technicians and volunteers are delivering AIDS care with grace, compassion and strength. If we are to meet the needs of our patients, we must understand better the skills that those providers are using. With this knowledge we can help increasing numbers of people find gratification and hope in this work' (Cooke, 1987).

In the same way that people with AIDS need to feel cared for and loved, so their lovers, companions, friends, nurses and doctors need the opportunity to share their own emotions. The sadness and anger that is felt whenever AIDS claims another patient, friend or loved one is an important part of the natural history of the disease – it should not simply be dismissed. Living with HIV infection and its various consequences is increasingly an issue for the entire community, and it is to the community as a whole that we must look for support and resources to help us through the difficult years that lie ahead.

References

Anon. (1987) *Taking a Break: a guide for people caring at home,* London, Health Education Authority/King's Fund.

Berkowitz, R. (1986) AIDS as identity, in M. Callen (ed) *PWA Coalition Newsline,* **15,** p 23–24.

Blachman, M. (1988) Seropositive women: clinical issues and approaches, *Focus,* **3, 3.**

Boyton, R. & Scambler, G. (1988) Survey of general practitioners' attitudes to AIDS in the North West Thames and East Anglian regions, *British Medical Journal,* **296,** p 538.

Cannadine, D. (1981) War and death, grief and mourning in modern Britain, in J. Whaley (ed) *Mirrors of Mortality: studies in the social history of death,* London, Europa.

Cooke, M. (1987) Learning to care: health care workers respond to AIDS, *Focus,* **2, 7.**

Crown, J. (1987) Planning services within the NHS. AIDS: planning local services, *King's Fund Project Paper,* 68, London, King's Fund.

Deitch, D. (1987) Counselling the HIV seropositive transfusion recipient, *Focus,* **2, 8.**

DE (1987) *AIDS and Employment,* London, Dept of Employment.

Frontliners (1987) *Living with AIDS: A guide to survival by people with AIDS,* Frontliners, London.

HMSO (1987) Third Report of the Social Services Committee of the House of Commons, *Problems Associated with AIDS,* 13 May, London, HMSO.

Jones, P. (1986) AIDS: planning for our future, *Social Work Today* 9 February, p 10.

Kohner, N. (1988) *Caring at Home: a handbook for people looking after someone at home — someone young or old, handicapped or disabled, ill or frail,* London, Health Education Authority/King's Fund.

Malcolmson, S. (1988) Sex and death in Key West, *Mother Jones* (Boston), February/March.

Newton, T. (1987) Opening Address: caring for people with AIDS in the community, DHSS/ King's Fund, London.

Platt, D. (1987) The community care challenge for local authorities in AIDS: planning local services, *King's Fund Project Paper,* 68, London, King's Fund.

Rayner, G. (1987) AIDS: future directions. AIDS: planning local services. *King's Fund Project Paper,* 41, London, King's Fund.

RIS (1987) *AIDS: The Issues for Housing,* London, Resource Information Service.

Russo, V. (1988) Coming out as a PWA to one's family, *PWA Coalition Newsline,* **30.**

Schofferman, J. (1987) Medicine and the psychology of treating the terminally ill, in L. McKusick (ed) *What to Do about AIDS: physicians and mental health professionals discuss the issues,* University of California Press, San Francisco.

Williams, S. (1987) (ed) *Caring for People with AIDS in the Community,* London DHSS/King's Fund.

Zachar, B. (1987) Depression busters, *PWA Coalition Newsline,* **15,** pp 23–24.

Appendix A

ADDITIONAL RESOURCES WITH AN EMPHASIS ON SEX AND SEXUALITY

The *Family Planning Association* runs courses on sex and personal relationships for teachers, health professionals and health educators. It also offers training programmes in the area of HIV infection and AIDS and has a wide range of relevant publications. Details from:
Family Planning Association
27–35 Mortimer Street
London W1N 7RJ
01-636 7866

The *International Planned Parenthood Federation* (IPPF) provides education, information and training on sex, contraception and personal relationships. Details from:
International Planned Parenthood Federation
Regent's College
Inner Circle
Regent's Park
London NW1 4NS

Brook Advisory Centres produce a variety of leaflets and information on sex and contraception. Their national network of centres offers advice and counselling to individuals. Details from:
Brook Advisory Centre
153a East Street
London SE17 2SD
01-708 1234

The *Women's Education Resource Centre* offers resources and materials relating to sex and sexuality. It publishes a magazine called *Gen*. Details from:
Women's Education Resource Centre
ILEA Drama and Tape Centre
Princeton Street
London WC1R 4BH

The *Women's Health and Reproductive Rights Information Centre* (WHRRIC) provides access to information and support, speakers and networks. Details from:

Women's Health and Reproductive Rights Information Centre
52 Featherstone Street
London EC1Y 8RT
01-251 6332

The *National Association of Young People's Counselling and Advisory Services* (NAYPCAS) offers information and access to a network of youth counselling agencies and annual training workshops. Details from:

National Association of Young People's Counselling and Advisory Services
17–23 Albion Street
Leicester LE1 6GD

The *National Youth Bureau* (NYB) can provide information and advice on a wide range of issues affecting young people, including sexuality and personal relationships. Details from:

National Youth Bureau
17–23 Albion Street
Leicester LE1 6GD

The *Lesbian and Gay Youth Movement* has details of local groups for young lesbians and young gay men. It also organises annual conferences. Details from:

Lesbian and Gay Youth Movement
BM GYM
London WC1N 3XX

The *Project for Advice, Counselling and Education* (PACE), based at the London Lesbian and Gay Centre, offers training in sexuality and sexual awareness. It also provides individual counselling. Details from:

Project for Advice, Counselling and Education
London Lesbian and Gay Centre
69 Cowcross Street
London EC1M 6BP
01-251 2689

Copies of *Fighting against Prejudice*, a training pack dealing with lesbian and gay issues, are available from:

NALGO
1 Mabledon Place
London WC1H 9AG

Copies of *Danger: Heterosexism at Work, Changing the World: a charter for gay and lesbian rights* and *Challenging Heterosexism in the Work Place: a training resource pack for personnel and training staff in local authorities* can be obtained from:
London Strategic Policy Unit
Publications Department
Middlesex House
20 Vauxhall Bridge Road
London SW1V 2SB

Copies of *Gay men at Work* and *All in a Day's Work: a report on anti-lesbian discrimination in London* can be obtained from:
Lesbian and Gay Employment Rights (LAGER)
Room 203
Southbank House
Black Prince Road
London SE1 7SJ

Useful books

Allen, I. (1986) *Education in Sex and Personal Relationships,* London, Policy Studies Institute.
Davies, M. (1985) *Sex Education for Young People with a Disability,* London, Association to Aid the Sexual and Personal Relationships of People with a Disability.
Dickson, A. (1985) *The Mirror Within,* London, Quartet Books.
Dixon, H. (1986) *Options for Change,* London, Family Planning Association Education Unit/British Institute of Mental Handicap Publications. (A staff training handbook on personal relationships and sexuality for people with a mental handicap.)
Heather, B. (1984) *Sharing,* London, Family Planning Association Education Unit.
Hughes, N. *et al.* (1984) *Stepping Out to Line: a workbook on lesbianism and feminism,* Press Gang Publishers.
Human Rights Foundation Inc. (1984) *Demystifying Homosexuality,* Philadelphia, Human Rights Foundation.
Massey, D. *et al* (1988) *Teaching about HIV and AIDS,* London, HEA.
National Youth Bureau (1987) *Windows on Practice: the youth service response to AIDS,* Leicester, National Youth Bureau.
Szirom, T. & Dyson, S. (1986) *Greater Expectations: a source book for working with girls and young women,* Wisbech, Learning Development Associates.

Trenchard, L. (ed) (1984) *Young Lesbians,* London, London Gay Teenage Group.

Trenchard, L. (ed) & Warren, H. (1985) *Talking about Youth Work,* London, London Gay Teenage Group.

Warren, H. (ed) (1984) *Talking about School,* London, London Gay Teenage Group.

Warren, H. & Trenchard, L. (eds) (1984) *Something to Tell You,* London, London Gay Teenage Group.

Appendix B

ADDITIONAL RESOURCES WITH AN EMPHASIS ON DRUG USE AND DRUGS EDUCATION

The *Teachers Advisory Council on Alcohol and Drugs Education* (TACADE) has produced a number of publications on health and drug education. Details from:
TACADE Publications
3rd Floor
Furness House
Trafford Road
Salford M5 2XJ

The *Health Education Authority* (HEA) has produced a resource list on drugs education. Details from:
Health Education Authority
Hamilton House
Mabledon Place
London WC1H 9TX

The *Standing Conference on Drug Abuse* (SCODA) has a range of publications of relevance to drugs education. Details from:
Standing Conference on Drug Abuse
1–4 Hatton Place
Hatton Gardens
London EC1N 8ND
01-430 2341

The *Institute for the Study of Drug Dependency* (ISDD) has a range of publications of relevance to drugs education. Details from:
Institute for the Study of Drug Dependency
1–4 Hatton Place
Hatton Gardens
London EC1N 8ND
01-430 1991

Drugs, Alcohol and Women Nationally (DAWN) can offer advice on women and drug use. Details from:
DAWN
Boundary House
91–93 Charterhouse Street
London EC1M 6HR
(01-250 3284)

A wide variety of health education resources are now available with an emphasis on drugs education. These include:

Free to Choose (1981) An approach to drug education for use with all ages in secondary schools. Salford, TACADE.

Facts and Feelings about Drugs but Decisions about Situations (1982) London, Institute for the Study of Drug Dependency.

Drinking Choices: Training Manual for Alcohol Educators (1983) Details from TACADE Publications.

Drugs Demystified (1984) Training pack. Institute for the Study of Drug Dependency.

WREAD (Work Related Education on Alcohol and Drugs) Pack (1985) London, Institute for the Study of Drug Dependency.

Drugs: Responding to the Challenge (1987) Materials for drug education and training. London, Health Education Authority.

Drug Wise (1987) Health education materials for 14–18-year-olds.
    Salford, TACADE.

The following resources address drugs education within the context of general education about health and personal relationships:

Choose Health (1987) Leicester/London, National Youth Bureau/Health Education Authority. Materials for work in youth clubs and work with young people.

Health Education Authority Health Action Pack: health education for 16–19s (1988) London, Health Education Authority. Health education materials for use with 16–19s. Details from: National Extension College, 18 Brooklands Avenue, Cambridge CB2 2HN

HEA Health Skills Manual (1988) A skills-based teaching manual for secondary schools. Details from: Jen Anderson, Counselling and Career Development Unit, University of Leeds, 22 Clarendon Place, Leeds LS2 9JY

HEA Secondary Schools Pack (1988) A pack which covers a variety of health topics and includes guidance on how to develop and co-ordinate health education in secondary schools. Details from: The Young People's Programme, Hamilton House, Mabledon Place, London WC1H 9TX.

Appendix C

ADDITIONAL RESOURCES FOR HEALTH EDUCATORS

Some useful addresses and telephone numbers

Terrence Higgins Trust – provides advice and counselling about HIV infection and AIDS; can also provide details about local AIDS helplines
  01-242 1010 (Monday–Friday, 7–10 pm, with answerphone service outside these hours)
  01-278 8745 (priority number for counselling and advice for those with HIV and AIDS)
  01-405 2381 (Wednesday, 7–10 pm, advice on legal issues affecting people with AIDS and HIV infection)

Body Positive – a support group providing counselling for people with HIV infection
  01-373 9124 (7–10 pm, seven days a week)

Frontliners – a support group for people with AIDS
  01-831 0330

Haemophilia Society
  01-928 2020

Positively Women – a London-based support group for women with HIV infection and AIDS
  Contact via Standing Conference on Drug Abuse (SCODA), see below

London Lighthouse – a London centre providing support and hospice care for people with HIV infection and AIDS
  01-221 6513

Standing Conference on Drug Abuse (SCODA)
  01-430 2341

Health Education Authority
  01-631 0930

London Lesbian and Gay Switchboard
01-837 7324 (24 hours, seven days a week)

National AIDS Helpline – provides advice and counselling for people worried about AIDS/HIV
0800-567123 (24 hours, seven days a week)

Scottish AIDS Monitor
031-557 1757

Welsh AIDS Monitor
0222-223443

Services for minority and ethnic groups

Cantonese
0800-282 446 (Tuesday, 6–10 pm)

Asian languages (Urdu, Hindi, Punjab, Gujerati, Bengali/Sylheti)
0800-282 445 (Wednesday, 6–10 pm)

Afro-Caribbean Service
0800-567 123 (Friday, 6–10 pm)

Some useful organisations

AVERT – a charitable organisation concerned with research and education about HIV infection and AIDS
0403-864010

London Friend – a support and befriending group for lesbians and gay men
01-837 3337 (7–10 pm)

Release – a service for drug users requiring legal advice
01-377 5905 (10 am–5 pm)
01-603 8654 (emergency number available 24 hours)

Black Community AIDS Team – a group which provides support and advice to meet black people's needs concerning HIV infection and AIDS

The Landmark, 47 Tulse Hill, London SW2 2TN

Drugline Drug Services – an organisation which provides information about the provision of services for drug users available around the country

Freephone 01-831 6738 (for the south of the country)

Freephone 01-242 9799 (for the north of the country)

Mainliners – an organisation which provides support groups for HIV-positive drug users and former drug users. Contact via the Terrence Higgins Trust

Some useful books and printed resources

Aggleton, P. & Homans, H. (eds) (1988) *Social Aspects of AIDS,* Lewes, Falmer Press.

Aggleton, P., Hart, G., Davies, P. (1989) *AIDS: Social Representations, Social Practices,* Lewes, Falmer Press

Altman, D. (1986) *AIDS and the New Puritanism,* London, Pluto Press.

Chirimuuta, R. C. and Chirimuuta, R. J. (1987) *AIDS, Africa and Racism.* Available from R. Chirimuuta, Bretby House, Stanhope, Bretby, nr Burton-on-Trent, Derbyshire DE15 0PT.

McKie, R. (1986) *Panic: The Story of AIDS,* London, Thorsons.

Miller, D. (1987) *Living with HIV and AIDS,* London, Macmillan.

Patton, C. (1985) *Sex and Germs – The Politics of AIDS,* Boston, South End Press.

Richardson, D. (1987) *Women and the AIDS Crisis,* London, Pandora Press.

Robertson, R. (1987) *Heroin, AIDS and Society,* London, Hodder & Stoughton.

Tatchell, P. (1987) *AIDS: a guide to survival,* London, Gay Men's Press.

Watney, S. (1987) *Policing Desire: pornography, AIDS and the media,* London, Methuen/Comedia.

Copies of the Health Education Authority's leaflet *Authoritative information about AIDS* lists AIDS titles published by the HEA. This can be obtained free from:

Health Education Authority
Hamilton House
Mabledon Place
London WC1H 9TX

Copies of the leaflet *Your Guide to Safer Sex and the Condom* and the factsheets *Some Laws on Sex* and *Sex Education in Schools* are available from:

Family Planning Information Service
27/35 Mortimer Street
London W1N 7RJ

Copies of the Health Education Authority *Resource List on AIDS* are available from:

Health Education Authority
Hamilton House
Mabledon Place
London WC1H 9TX

Copies of the leaflet *AIDS - how drug users can avoid it* are available from:
SCODA
1–4 Hatton Place
Hatton Gardens
London EC1N 8ND

Copies of the booklet *Children at School and Problems Related to AIDS,* produced for teachers by the Department of Education and Science, can be obtained free from:
Publications Despatch Centre
Canons Park
Middlesex HA7 1AZ

Copies of the booklet *AIDS and Employment,* produced by the Department of Employment and the Health & Safety Executive, can be obtained free from:
The Mailing House
Leeland Road
London W13 9HL

Copies of *AIDS in Employment,* a statement produced jointly by the TUC, the CBI and ACAS, can be obtained free from:
TUC Publications
Congress House
Great Russell Street
London WC1B 3LS

Details of *AIDS - a TUC course,* a training pack for trade unionists, can be obtained from:
TUC Publications
Congress House
Great Russell Street
London WC1B 3LS

Copies of *Educating about AIDS – a discussion document for community physicians, health education officers, health advisers and others with a responsibility for education about AIDS* can be obtained free from:
Sara Marshall
National Health Service Training Authority
St Bartholomew Court
18 Christmas Steps
Bristol BS1 5BT
0272-291029

A subscription to the *AIDS Newsletter*, a monthly update on medical, scientific and social issues, can be taken out by writing to:
Bureau of Hygiene and Tropical Diseases
Keppel Street
London WC1E 7HT

A subscription to *Focus: a guide to AIDS research*, a monthly publication from the AIDS Health Project at the University of California, San Francisco, can be taken out by writing to:
AIDS Health Project
UCSF
Box 0884
San Francisco
CA 94143-0884
USA

An extensive list of health education materials produced by the Terrence Higgins Trust is available from:
The Terrence Higgins Trust
BM AIDS
London WC1N 3XX

A leaflet called *AIDS and Childbirth* can be obtained from:
AVERT
PO Box 91
Horsham
West Sussex RH13 7YR

Index